Walter Bockting, PhD
Eric Avery, MD
Editors

Transgender Health and HIV Prevention: Needs Assessment Studies from Transgender Communities Across the United States

Transgender Health and HIV Prevention: Needs Assessment Studies from Transgender Communities Across the United States has been co-published simultaneously as *International Journal of Transgenderism*, Volume 8, Numbers 2/3 2005.

Pre-publication REVIEWS, COMMENTARIES, EVALUATIONS . . .

"**I** HIGHLY RECOMMEND THIS BOOK to everyone who works with the transgender population or who wishes to understand more fully the lives and experiences of this increasingly visible population. Generally, work about transgender people is confined to males-to-females but this book is equally inclusive of the lives and issues of females-to-males. It shares information from critical needs assessments on how transgender people may be served in the widest possible way."

Ronni L. Sanlo, EdD
Director
UCLA Lesbian Gay Bisexual
Transgender Center

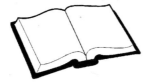

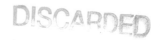

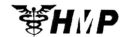

The Haworth Medical Press®
An Imprint of The Haworth Press, Inc.

Transgender Health
and HIV Prevention:
Needs Assessment Studies
from Transgender Communities
Across the United States

Transgender Health and HIV Prevention: Needs Assessment Studies from Transgender Communities Across the United States has been co-published simultaneously as *International Journal of Transgenderism*, Volume 8, Numbers 2/3 2005.

Monographic Separates from the *International Journal of Transgenderism*™

For additional information on these and other Haworth Press titles, including descriptions, tables of contents, reviews, and prices, use the QuickSearch catalog at http://www.HaworthPress.com.

Transgender Health and HIV Prevention: Needs Assessment Studies from Transgender Communities Across the United States, edited by Walter Bockting, PhD, and Eric Avery, MD (Vol. 8, No. 2/3, 2005). *"I highly recommend this book to everyone who works with the transgender population or who wishes to understand more fully the lives and experiences of this increasingly visible population." (Ronni L. Sanlo, EdD, Director, UCLA Lesbian Gay Bisexual Transgender Center)*

Transgender Health and HIV Prevention: Needs Assessment Studies from Transgender Communities Across the United States

Walter Bockting, PhD
Eric Avery, MD
Editors

Transgender Health and HIV Prevention: Needs Assessment Studies from Transgender Communities Across the United States has been co-published simultaneously as *International Journal of Transgenderism*, Volume 8, Numbers 2/3 2005.

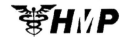

The Haworth Medical Press®
An Imprint of The Haworth Press, Inc.

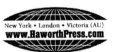

New York • London • Victoria (AU)
www.HaworthPress.com

Published by

The Haworth Medical Press®, 10 Alice Street, Binghamton, NY 13904-1580 USA

The Haworth Medical Press® is an imprint of The Haworth Press, Inc., 10 Alice Street, Binghamton, NY 13904-1580 USA.

Transgender Health and HIV Prevention: Needs Assessment Studies from Transgender Communities Across the United States has been co-published simultaneously as *International Journal of Transgenderism*™, Volume 8, Numbers 2/3 2005.

Cover credit: Linoleum Block Prints by Eric Avery <http://www.DocArt.com>. Used with permission.

Cover design by Jennifer M. Gaska.

Library of Congress Cataloging-in-Publication Data

Bockting, Walter O.
Transgender health and HIV prevention : needs assessment studies from transgender communities across the United States / Walter Bockting ; Eric Avery, editor.
      p. cm.
    "Transgender health and HIV prevention: needs assessment studies from transgender communities across the United States has been co-published simultaneously as International Journal of Transgenderism, volume 8, numbers 2/3, 2005."
    Includes bibliographical references and index.
    ISBN-13: 978-0-7890-3015-3 (pkb. : alk. paper)
    ISBN-10: 0-7890-3015-2 (pkb. : alk. paper)
    1. AIDS (Disease)–United States–Prevention. 2. AIDS (Disease)–Risk factors–United States. 3. Transsexuals–Health and hygiene–United States. 4. Transsexuals–Sexual behavior–United States. I. Avery, Eric. II. Title.
RA643.83.B63 2005
362.196'9792'00866–dc22
                                                        2005015577

Indexing, Abstracting & Website/Internet Coverage

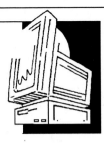

This section provides you with a list of major indexing & abstracting services and other tools for bibliographic access. That is to say, each service began covering this periodical during the year noted in the right column. Most Websites which are listed below have indicated that they will either post, disseminate, compile, archive, cite, or alert their own Website users with research-based content from this work. (This list is as current as the copyright date of this publication.)

Abstracting, Website/Indexing Coverage ....Year When Coverage Began

- *British Journal of Psychotherapy* 2005
- *CareData: the database supporting social care management and practice*
  <http://www.elsc.org.uk/caredata/caredata.htm> 2005
- *CINAHL (Cumulative Index to Nursing & Allied Health Literature), in print, EBSCO,*
  and SilverPlatter, DataStar, and PaperChase. (Support materials include Subject
  Heading List, Database Search Guide, and instructional video.)
  <http://www.cinahl.com> 2005
- *EBSCOhost Electronic Journals Service (EJS) <http://ejournals.ebsco.com>* 2005
- *Family Index Database <http://www.familyscholar.com>* 2005
- *GLBT Life (EBSCO Publishing) <http://www.epnet.com/academic/glbt.asp>* 2005
- *Google <http://www.google.com>* 2004
- *Google Scholar <http://scholar.google.com>* 2004
- *Haworth Document Delivery Center <http://www.HaworthPress.com/journals/dds.asp>* .. 2004
- *HOMODOK/"Relevant" Bibliographic database, Documentation Centre for Gay &*
  Lesbian Studies, University of Amsterdam (selective printed abstracts in "Homologie"
  and bibliographic computer databases covering cultural, historical, social & political
  aspects) <http://www.ihlia.nl/> 2004
- *Links@Ovid (via CrossRef targeted DOI links) <http://www.ovid.com>* 2005
- *OCLC Public Affairs Information Service <http://www.pais.org>* 2004
- *Ovid Linksolver (OpenURL link resolver via CrossRef targeted DOI Links)*
  <http://www.linksolver.com> 2005
- *Referativnyi Zhurnal (Abstracts Journal of the All-Russian Institute of Scientific*
  and Technical Information–in Russian) <http://www.viniti.ru> 2005
- *Social Services Abstracts <http://www.csa.com>* 2004
- *Social Work Abstracts <http://www.silverplatter.com/catalog/swab.htm>* 2005
- *SocioAbs <http://www.csa.com>* 2004
- *Sociological Abstracts (SA) <http://www.csa.com>* 2004
- *Studies on Women and Gender Abstracts <http://www.tandf.co.uk/swa>* 2005

(continued)

Special Bibliographic Notes related to special journal issues
[separates] and indexing/abstracting:

- indexing/abstracting services in this list will also cover material in any "separate" that is co-published simultaneously with Haworth's special thematic journal issue or DocuSerial. Indexing/abstracting usually covers material at the article/chapter level.
- monographic co-editions are intended for either non-subscribers or libraries which intend to purchase a second copy for their circulating collections.
- monographic co-editions are reported to all jobbers/wholesalers/approval plans. The source journal is listed as the "series" to assist the prevention of duplicate purchasing in the same manner utilized for books-in-series.
- to facilitate user/access services all indexing/abstracting services are encouraged to utilize the co-indexing entry note indicated at the bottom of the first page of each article/chapter/contribution.
- this is intended to assist a library user of any reference tool (whether print, electronic, online, or CD-ROM) to locate the monographic version if the library has purchased this version but not a subscription to the source journal.
- individual articles/chapters in any Haworth publication are also available through the Haworth Document Delivery Service (HDDS).

Transgender Health and HIV Prevention: Needs Assessment Studies from Transgender Communities Across the United States

CONTENTS

ABOUT THE EDITORS

Walter Bockting, PhD, is Licensed Psychologist and Associate Professor at the Program in Human Sexuality, Department of Family Medicine and Community Health, University of Minnesota Medical School, Minneapolis, Minnesota, USA. He is also on the graduate faculty of the University's Center for Advanced Feminist Studies, and he coordinates the University of Minnesota Transgender Health Services, integrating clinical service, education, and research to promote the health and well-being of the transgender community. Dr. Bockting is a native from The Netherlands and received his PhD from the Vrije Universiteit in Amsterdam. His research interests include transgender identity, sexuality and the Internet, the prevention of HIV and other sexually-transmitted diseases, and the promotion of sexual health. He has been the recipient of grants from the American Foundation for AIDS Research, the Sisters of Mercy, the Minnesota Department of Health, and the National Institutes of Health. Dr. Bockting is the author of many scientific articles and editor of *Gender Dysphoria: Interdisciplinary Approaches in Clinical Management* (The Haworth Press, Inc., 1992), *Transgender and HIV: Risks, Prevention, and Care* (The Haworth Press, Inc., 2001), and *Masturbation as a Means of Achieving Sexual Health* (The Haworth Press, Inc., 2002). He serves on the editorial board of the *Journal of Psychology & Human Sexuality* and the *Journal of Homosexuality* and is a member of the Board of Directors of the Harry Benjamin International Gender Dysphoria Association. Dr. Bockting is the 2005 President of the Society for the Scientific Study of Sexuality.

Eric Avery, MD, is Associate Professor of Clinical Psychiatry at the University of Texas Medical Branch in Galveston, Texas. He is also the Director of HIV Psychiatric Services for the University as well as an Associate Member of the Institute for Medical Humanities and an Associate Member of the Graduate Faculty for the School of Biomedical Sciences. He has been with the UTMB HIV Clinic since 1982. He received his Doctorate of Medicine and completed a one-year internship in the Department of Psychiatry at UTMB before transferring to New York State Psychiatric Institute where he completed three more years of residency in General Psychiatry. In 1994, he completed a fellowship in Consultation & Liaison Psychiatry for HIV/AIDS. In 1985, he began working with HIV+ transsexuals. In 1999, he helped open the Gender Identity Clinic at UTMB. In 1997, he presented a paper, "International Transgender Surgeon Survey and Gender Identity Disorder Clinic Surveys," at the XV Harry Benjamin International Symposium that resulted in a change in the HBIGDA Standards of Care addressing access to care for transsexuals with HIV. Dr. Avery also serves on the Editorial Board of the Medical Humanities Review at UTMB. He is also a world-renown visual artist. He has received numerous honors for his artistic works, which include permanent collections and exhibitions, displayed on local, national, and international levels. His artwork can be viewed on his website: www.DocArt.com.

Dedication to Mikki Jackson

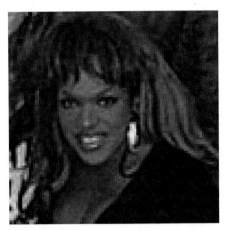

October 1971-October 2003

This collection of original research on Transgender Health and HIV prevention is dedicated to the memory and spirit of Mikki Jackson. Mikki was a male-to-female transsexual who lived life to the fullest. She was loved by most people who knew her, envied by some for her natural beauty, and feared by others for her sharp tongue and strong personality. Mikki was one of my dearest friends. She was there for me as a guide and source of confidence and support as I tentatively came out as being transgender to my family and friends. Since Mikki has made the transition from a material existence to a spiritual one, I have had a difficult time mourning her death. I attended her memorial service and made the perfunctory comments that one would expect from a best friend, but I never shed a tear. In November of 2004, I was in attendance at an historic Transgender Consultation convened to give the officials at the Center for Disease Control and Prevention (CDC) in Atlanta, Georgia, a better understanding of the unique aspects of the transgender population. While there, I publicly acknowledged her death

and requested a moment of silence to which the audience of some fifty transgender community activists, healthcare professionals, and CDC representatives respectfully complied, but, as before, I could not bring forth any tears for my departed friend. The following month, at the ninth installment of the All Gender Health Seminar (an intervention designed by and for Minnesota's transgender community), I dedicated the event to the memory and spirit of Mikki, but still no tears.

As I write this dedication, I ask myself: Why? Why can't I allow myself to be visibly moved by the early passing of one of my dearest and closet friends? Maybe it is because of the way she died, frail and ravaged by the devastating effects of AIDS. Or perhaps it is because I have lost so many friends and family members to the disease; including my own father.

Mikki lived a painful existence. Born to an African American father and Native American mother, she was instantly exposed to the prejudice and discrimination that people of color endure in America. Like many transgender persons, she recognized her femininity at a very early age. Being a feminine boy contributed to Mikki's leaving her family's home at the age of 12, and she found herself on her own without the skills to cope with her internal anguish and the harsh reality of trying to provide for the basic necessities of life: food, shelter and clothing. Survival sex became a way of life for her. She told me many stories of being abused by older men, being used like a blow-up sex doll for their pleasure. Mikki was a naturally beautiful girl, no plastic surgery, no hormones or silicone. A man could walk hand in hand with her down the street and no one would ever suspect that she was born male. Mikki began to use her beauty as a weapon. She would lure men into her tangled web and then she would turn the tables on them. Many men thought she would be the receptive partner, but Mikki would have none of it. If she couldn't be the "top," then it wasn't happening. She practiced her own form of "safe" sex. It wasn't about protecting her *physical* health, but rather her *emotional* health.

Mikki was one of the most intelligent persons I have ever known. A gifted visual artist, she created wonderful collages and paintings. She was a clothing designer, taking everyday articles of clothing and turning them into sexy ensembles that many Hollywood starlets would envy. Her hairstyling skills were employed by some of the most popular drag queen performers in Minneapolis. But her formal education was stunted at an early age. She dropped out of high school before completing the ninth grade, because of the bullying from classmates that proved to be too much for her to bear. She was repeatedly fired from gainful employment upon discovery of her transgender status.

Unfortunately, Mikki's story is not atypical. In fact, it is quite common for transgender women of color. On the street at an early age, involved in sex work, with drugs and alcohol as medication. Medication for the discomfort they experience from living in the wrong body, and the abuse they suffer because of it. The lives of transgender women of color constitutes a subculture within a subculture; a group with its own language, rules and hierarchy. Theirs is a risky life, filled with violence, addiction, and disease, including HIV and other sexually transmitted infections. However, there are no specific, comprehensive intervention models for the Mikki's of the world. When it comes to HIV prevention interventions, these unique women are all too often left out in the cold. They don't fit neatly in either gender category; not fully male or female, their lives remain invisible, un-noticed and un-appreciated.

Mikki, like many transsexuals and transgender individuals, was conflicted about her gender identity. She would constantly vacillate back and forth between her male persona and female persona. She simultaneously thought that God was punishing her and blessing her with these transgender feelings. I know that many of my transgender sisters and brothers feel the same way. I sometimes feel that way myself. So while it has been difficult for me to shed tears for this beautiful and tender soul, it saddens me deeply to know that this cycle will continue until our community rises up and screams at the top of our collective lungs: Enough! Perhaps then, law makers, healthcare officials and other concerned allies will recognize the humanity of our lives and create some solutions for the leviathan problems of unemployment, homelessness, addiction, and HIV infection experienced by so many in this population. Until then, we will continue to posthumously dedicate publications and events to the memory of transgender individuals who succumb to this opportunistic virus.

Even though Mikki's death certificate clearly indicated that she died from complications of AIDS, I know the truth. She died from benign neglect, loneliness, and societal contempt. I still love you, Mikki, and all those like you. Rest in peace.

Darling Mikki

before the morphine kicked in
before the commute was two
and a half hours and pneumonia
was a semi-annual calamity

all the way back
before you made all the
men horney, before they figured
out that you were a top, and
liked being in control

before the leaves turned red and
gold on the tree that was your life,
before lonely was attached to your soul
anchoring you to your bed

before the sores took over your
body and your face and pain was your
constant companion, before you
cut off all friends who loved you.

You were a star/everyone knew it/
But you.

Andrea Jenkins, MS

Andrea Jenkins is a writer and poet living in Minneapolis, Minnesota. She is currently the Acting Coordinator of All Gender Health, a transgender-specific HIV/STI prevention program at the University of Minnesota. She is also a non-profit consultant specializing in organizational development and effectiveness. She can be reached at *shesgotgame1@msn.com.*

Photograph used with permission.

Introduction

HIV and AIDS continue to move through the fault lines in society, infecting some of our most marginalized populations. In order to respond to the pandemic with prevention and treatment, researchers have focused on identifying and studying these marginalized and disproportionately affected groups of people in order to develop HIV prevention programs. One of these marginalized groups is the transgender population.

Since completion of the first edited special journal issue and volume, *Transgender and HIV* (W. Bockting & S. Kirk, *International Journal of Transgenderism*, 3(1/2), 1999 [available at *www.symposion.com/ijt*] simultaneously published by The Haworth Press, Inc., 2001), a second generation of needs assessment studies were conducted in transgender communities across the United States. These studies broadened the assessment of needs to include the larger problems of social stigma, discrimination, and lack of access to transgender-specific and sensitive health care. This reflects the fact that HIV is often not the first priority for transgender individuals. In order for HIV prevention to be effective, a multitude of other issues such as gender dysphoria, mental health, substance abuse, housing, and employment, need to be addressed. The papers in this volume present the findings of these broader needs assessment studies, all of which were conducted by transgender community members in partnership with scientists in HIV prevention and public health. Study sites included San Francisco, Washington, DC, Philadelphia, Chicago, Houston, Boston, New England, San Juan, and Minneapolis/St. Paul.

We dedicate this collective work to the memory of Mikki Jackson. Mikki served on the advisory board of All Gender Health, an HIV prevention program in Minnesota that addresses transgender people's risk for HIV and other sexually transmitted infections in the light of their overall sexual health. Andrea Jenkins eloquently describes how Mikki's story is an example of how HIV infection of transgender individuals is embedded in an overall picture of marginalization and disenfranchisement.

Nemoto and colleagues from the Center for AIDS Prevention Studies at the University of California share the findings of focus groups and survey interviews with over 300 male-to-female transgender persons of color in San Francisco. They document the health and social services needs of African-Americans, Latinas, and Asian/Pacific Islanders in a city historically known as welcoming of sexual diversity. Although utilization rates of basic health care services were high, the use of social services, substance abuse treatment, psychological counseling, and gender transition-related medical services was low. Qualitative findings indicated that, even in a city as open to sexual diversity as San Francisco, transgender-specific programs and provider trainings were urgently needed on such issues as hormone use, gender role transition, HIV prevention and care, substance abuse, and mental health problems. Demonstrating the value of this research to study participants, Nemoto and his colleagues are

[Haworth co-indexing entry note]: "Introduction." Bockting, Walter, and Eric Avery. Co-published simultaneously in *International Journal of Transgenderism* (The Haworth Medical Press, an imprint of The Haworth Press, Inc.) Vol. 8, No. 2/3, 2005, pp. 1-3; and: *Transgender Health and HIV Prevention: Needs Assessment Studies from Transgender Communities Across the United States* (ed: Walter Bockting, and Eric Avery) The Haworth Medical Press, an imprint of The Haworth Press, Inc., 2005, pp. 1-3. Single or multiple copies of this article are available for a fee from The Haworth Document Delivery Service [1-800-HAWORTH, 9:00 a.m. - 5:00 p.m. (EST). E-mail address: docdelivery@haworthpress.com].

currently collaborating with other organizations in the Bay Area to address these important needs.

Also in San Francisco, Coan and colleagues explored the possible sources for the high rates of HIV infection among the city's male-to-female transgender population. On the basis of focus groups with transgender women and individual interviews with their male sexual partners, this study found that these male partners are of diverse socioeconomic backgrounds and sexual orientations, that drug use appears to play a role in unsafe sex, and that the male partners represent a possible bridge for HIV transmission among different populations given that they also reported sex with nontransgender women and men. Finally, they also found that men may engage more often in receptive anal sex with male-to-female transgender persons than they would admit. This study exposed the urgent need for HIV prevention strategies targeting the male partners of transgender persons.

Xavier and colleagues conducted an extensive needs assessment of about 250 transgender persons in Washington, DC. The HIV prevalence in their sample was 25%, and HIV positive status was predicted by being male-to-female (as opposed to female-to-male), a history of sexual assault and substance abuse, and unemployment. Knowledge of the Harry Benjamin International Gender Dysphoria Association's Standards of Care that guide access to hormone therapy and sex reassignment surgery was extremely low, especially among participants of color. Illicit hormone use and silicone injections were common. Employment, housing, and job training were the most commonly-reported immediate needs. Recommendations include vocational training and improving access to transgender-specific health and prevention services.

Kenagy and colleague conducted needs assessment studies in both Philadelphia and Chicago. Kenagy shares the process of involving members of the Philadelphia transgender community in the development of the survey instrument. About half of the largely African American study participants (male-to-female and female-to-male) reported having attempted suicide. High levels of violence were reported, particularly among male-to-females. Health and social service needs included job training and employment, health and dental care, legal services, education, and counseling. In Chicago, 14% of 111 participants reported being HIV positive. They were all male-to-female and the majority was of color. Again, participants experienced high levels of physical and sexual violence, and in this sample, two-thirds had thought of attempting suicide. In Chicago, needed services included family planning, child care, and substance abuse treatment.

In Houston, Risser and colleagues assessed the risk behaviors of male-to-female transgender persons (N = 67) to inform the Community Planning Group in setting HIV prevention priorities. They found high rates of HIV infection (27%), and high prevalence of risky behaviors (unprotected sex and drug use), intimate partner violence, and suicidal ideation.

Sperber and colleagues examined the health needs of transgender people in Boston. They also assessed the experiences of transgender and transsexual individuals with the existing health care system. Findings from focus groups indicated that ignorance, insensitivity, and discrimination appeared to be the norm. This included providers' refusal to treat transgender persons, lack of respect for preferred pronouns, lack of knowledge about transgender-specific care, and focus on transgender issues when these are not paramount. The authors conclude that the need for provider training is imminent.

Lurie provides such training in the New England area. He interviewed providers of HIV-related care and advocacy on their knowledge and experience in working with transgender people. Providers reported a desire to treat transgender clients respectfully, but also admitted to a lack of comfort, knowledge, and skills. Providers complained of having inadequate time to build trusting relationships with their clients and a lack of evidence-based treatment protocols. The results of this study inform the development of provider training that will increase access and the effectiveness of care.

Rodríguez-Madera and colleague offer an analysis of how prevailing gender norms impact the sexual and HIV risk behaviors of male-to-female transgender persons. Using data from questionnaires and in-depth interviews with members of the transgender community in San Juan, Puerto Rico, the authors argue that traditional notions of femininity undermine the negotiation of safer sex for transgender persons, as they do for nontransgender women in Latin societies. The authors recommend that these notions of femininity be addressed in HIV prevention interventions. In addition, social vulnerability and institutional exclusion were identified as barriers to effective HIV prevention.

Finally, Bockting and colleagues compared the HIV risks and health issues of transgender people (male-to-female and female-to-male) in Minnesota with two other sexual minorities in Minneapolis/St. Paul: men who have sex with men, and women who have sex with women and men. Baseline data of interventions that reached a total of 809 participants showed no differences in overall sexual risk behavior between the three groups. Transgender persons were less likely to have multiple partners and more likely to be monogamous than men who have sex with men; no differences were found between transgender persons and the women in this respect. Only one transgender person reported being HIV positive (compared to 17% of the men). This is in contrast with the high HIV prevalence rates reported in many of the other studies in this collection; the possible reasons for this discrepancy are discussed. Consistent with the other studies, transgender persons were the most likely to report depression and suicidal ideation, and reported the lowest levels of social support. The authors conclude that the role of gender in HIV risk needs to be accounted for in targeted HIV prevention efforts.

Together, these studies confirm that, also within the transgender population, women of color–particularly those with the least economic and social power–appear at especially high risk for HIV infection and transmission. In addition, male partners of male-to-female transgender persons emerged as a high risk group in need of prevention research and education. Although female-to-male transgender persons appear less affected by HIV, the risk of particu-larly female-to-males who have sex with men should not be ignored. Despite the demonstrated need, access to appropriate HIV prevention and care remains extremely limited. Moreover, the broader health and social service needs of transgender communities across the United States and its territories are vast. The need for provider training is imminent. Recurring findings across the studies in this volume include widespread mental health concerns and the need for help with employment, housing, and substance abuse. Finally, participants reported high levels of violence, an issue that becomes even more poignant in light of a series of hate crimes and murders perpetrated against transgender persons across the country (see *http://www.gender.org/remember/day*). We cannot remain silent and do nothing.

We would like to express our gratitude to the many transgender study participants who gave generously of their time and energy to make greater understanding of the needs of transgender people possible. It's now up to all of us to answer the call for intervention and research to address these needs and promote transgender people's health and well-being.

Walter Bockting, PhD
Eric Avery, MD
Editors

ACKNOWLEDGMENTS

The Editors would like to thank Noelle Gray, MPH, Managing Editor of the *International Journal of Transgenderism*, for her assistance with the review of manuscripts, communication with authors, and preparation of the final manuscript for publication. Preliminary versions of several papers in this volume were presented in a plenary symposium at the 2001 biennial conference of the Harry Benjamin International Gender Dysphoria Association in Galveston, Texas. We acknowledge the financial support from the U.S. Surgeon General's Leadership Campaign on AIDS for that symposium.

Health and Social Services for Male-to-Female Transgender Persons of Color in San Francisco

Tooru Nemoto, PhD
Don Operario, PhD
JoAnne Keatley, MSW

SUMMARY. This article presents findings from an investigation of health needs, service utilization, and perceived barriers to services among male-to-female (MtF) transgender persons of color in San Francisco. Focus groups (n = 48) and survey interviews (n = 332) were conducted with convenience samples recruited from the community. Participants reported a range of health and social services needed during the previous year, with African-Americans and Latinas showing particularly strong service needs. Rates of utilizing services were high for basic health care but lower for social services, substance abuse treatment, psychological counseling, and gender transition-related medical services. No significant ethnic group differences in health service utilization were found. Qualitative findings evinced the call for transgender-specific programs and advanced provider training on transgender issues such as hormone use, gender transition, HIV/ AIDS care and prevention, substance abuse, and mental health problems. *[Article copies available for a fee from The Haworth Document Delivery Service: 1-800-HAWORTH. E-mail address: <docdelivery@haworthpress.com> Website: <http://www.HaworthPress.com> © 2005 by The Haworth Press, Inc. All rights reserved.]*

KEYWORDS. Transgender, services utilization, gender transition, drug use, mental health

INTRODUCTION

San Francisco has historically been a welcoming environment for diverse sexual communities including transgender persons, gay men, and lesbians. Driven by grassroots efforts, the city has advanced measures for the protection of civil and legal rights for sexual and gender mi-

Tooru Nemoto, PhD, Don Operario, PhD, and JoAnne Keatley, MSW, all are affiliated with the University of California San Francisco, Center for AIDS Prevention Studies, San Francisco, CA.

Address correspondence to: Tooru Nemoto, PhD, Universty of California San Francisco, Center for AIDS Prevention Studies, Suite 600, 74 New Montgomery Street, San Francisco, CA 94105 USA (E-mail: tnemoto@ psg.ucsf.edu).

The authors would like to thank everyone who assisted in the research study and the implementation of the community intervention project, including the study participants, community collaborators, outreach workers, health educators, and health professionals who provide services to MtF transgender persons of color.

The study was supported in part by the Substance Abuse and Mental Health Services Administration (Grants No.: H79-TI12592 and U97-SM53769), and the National Institutes on Drug Abuse (Grant No.: R01 DA11589).

Points of view and opinions expressed in the manuscript are not those of the government agencies.

[Haworth co-indexing entry note]: "Health and Social Services for Male-to-Female Transgender Persons of Color in San Francisco." Nemoto, Tooru, Don Operario, and JoAnne Keatley. Co-published simultaneously in *International Journal of Transgenderism* (The Haworth Medical Press, an imprint of The Haworth Press, Inc.) Vol. 8, No. 2/3, 2005, pp. 5-19; and: *Transgender Health and HIV Prevention: Needs Assessment Studies from Transgender Communities Across the United States* (ed: Walter Bockting, and Eric Avery) The Haworth Medical Press, an imprint of The Haworth Press, Inc., 2005, pp. 5-19. Single or multiple copies of this article are available for a fee from The Haworth Document Delivery Service [1-800-HAWORTH, 9:00 a.m. - 5:00 p.m. (EST). E-mail address: docdelivery@haworthpress.com].

doi:10.1300/J485v08n02_02

norities such as non-discrimination in housing and employment, health care benefits for domestic partners, and public health services. In 2001, a landmark ordinance was passed making San Francisco the only city in the U.S. to cover city employees' expenses for sex reassignment surgery. San Francisco has been at the forefront of providing services to transgender persons compared to other parts of the U.S. However, the city's male-to-female (MtF) transgender population has remained at highest risk for HIV infection, substance abuse, and other adverse health outcomes (Clements-Nolle et al., 2001; Nemoto et al., 1999; 2004a, 2004b). This article explores the state of health and social services for San Francisco's MtF transgender community using findings from a quantitative survey and a focus group study of life experiences among MtF transgender persons.

Alarming Levels of HIV, Drug Abuse, and Mental Health Needs

According to the San Francisco Department of Public Health (SFDPH), the prevalence of HIV and substance abuse in the San Francisco transgender community has reached overwhelming levels (SFDPH, 1999). In a study of 392 MtF transgender persons, over one-third (35%) of the sample tested positive for HIV (SFDPH, 1999). Another study of MtF transgender persons in San Francisco found 48% were HIV positive (Nemoto et al., 1999). Moreover, an SFDPH executive report concluded, "Transgendered persons have been recently identified as a population that has been most severely affected by the HIV/AIDS epidemic" (SFDPH, 1998).

Drug use presents one of the most formidable risk behaviors for HIV transmission in this community. One-third of 296 MtF transgender persons seeking health care at a San Francisco clinic reported lifetime injection drug use (Zevin, 2000). Similarly, Nemoto et al. (1999) found 28% of a MtF transgender sample ever used drugs by injection, and 22% ever had a steady sex partner who injected drugs. In the SFDPH transgender risk behavior study (1999), the majority of the sample reported a history of non-injection drug use, including marijuana (90%), cocaine (66%), speed (57%), LSD (52%), poppers (50%), crack (48%), and heroin (24%).

About one-third (34%) reported a history of injection drug use (IDU) and, among them, 47% shared syringes with someone else, 49% used someone else's syringe to load their own drugs, and 29% shared cookers with someone else (SFDPH, 1999).

A complex network of psychological, socioeconomic, and cultural forces underlie HIV risk and drug abuse within the transgender community. As early as childhood, many MtF transgender persons experience high rates of rejection from family and peers, as well as feelings of alienation and hopelessness (Gagne et al., 1997; Kreiss and Patterson, 1997; Verschoor and Poortinga, 1988). Societal bias and stigmatization can lead to psychological vulnerability for MtF transgender persons, such as depression and increased suicidal ideation and attempts (Bockting, 1997; Cole et al., 2000). Negative psychosocial consequences might be heightened among MtF transgender persons of color, who experience the cumulative effects of racism and transgender stigma similar to minority homosexual men (Diaz, 1998). Because poverty and unemployment abound in the transgender community (Nemoto et al., 1999; Springer, 1999), commercial sex work can become an economic necessity for many MtF transgender persons who often cannot obtain or find work due to discrimination and limited job training opportunities (Elifson et al., 1993). To cope with the adversity of sex work, stigmatization, and daily life struggles, many MtF transgender persons resort to drug use (Bockting et al., 1998).

The Transgender Resources and Neighborhood Space (TRANS) project has been operated by our UCSF transgender health educators and researchers since October 2001. TRANS provides health promotion workshops, support groups, and referral services for both MtF and FtM transgender persons, as well as gender variant individuals at a safe space located at the Tenderloin district. The effectiveness of TRANS in the first three years was evaluated (Nemoto et al., 2005).

Local Responses to the Public Health Needs of the MtF Transgender Community

A number of efforts have sought to address health adversities facing San Francisco's MtF transgender community. Most notable is "Transgender Tuesday" at the Tom Waddell Clinic, a city public health clinic offering primary care, mental health, and social services for individuals who identify as transgender (MtF and FtM) or intersex. In addition, the Castro-Mission Health Center, another city clinic, runs the "Dimensions Program," targeting health needs of gay, lesbian, transgender, and intersex adolescents.

Community-based organizations have spearheaded the effort to improve transgender health in San Francisco, with a primary focus on HIV prevention. These include the Asian and Pacific Islander Wellness Center, Proyecto Contra SIDA por Vida, Ark of Refuge, and Tenderloin AIDS Resource Center, all of which collaborated in our research. Services provided by these community organizations and city clinics have filled critical gaps in transgender health care. As a result, transgender persons continue to migrate to San Francisco seeking basic rights and services. However, the work remains limited by insufficient funding, staff training and knowledge of transgender issues, and scant evaluation and research on transgender health services. Lombardi (2001) has argued that transgender persons require enhanced and specific services to mitigate health disparities facing the community, and that additional awareness, training, and medical resources for professionals working with transgender persons are necessary.

Study Goals

We conducted a study to investigate the social, psychological, and cultural context and determinants of HIV risk and drug use behaviors among transgender persons of color (African-Americans, Latinas, and Asian/Pacific Islanders) in San Francisco. Study results regarding substance abuse and HIV risk behaviors are published elsewhere (Nemoto et al., 2004a; 2004b). Access to and utilization of health and social services represent an important facet of the current study. We sought to identify and describe how health and social services respond to the unique needs of the MtF transgender community, particularly transgender persons of color. Two specific questions guide the study:

1. What are the health and social service needs of MtF transgender persons of color in San Francisco?
2. How do MtF transgender persons of color perceive the health and social services available to them?

METHOD

The research reported here was conducted in two phases. Phase one consisted of focus groups conducted between November 1999 and February 2000 with members of the MtF transgender community, which was used to guide the development of quantitative survey instruments for an epidemiological study. Phase two consisted of individual survey interviews, using the transgender-specific instruments, with a community sample of MtF transgender persons of color conducted between November, 2000, and July, 2001. Study methods are described elsewhere (Nemoto et al., 2004a; 2004b).

Participants

Participants were recruited using convenience sampling via outreach at venues in the community with high concentrations of MtF transgender persons and through referrals from the collaborating agencies. To be eligible, participants had to be MtF transgender (either pre- or post-operative status), 18 years or older, a person of color (African-American, Latina, or Asian/Pacific Islander), and have a history of commercial sex work.

In the first phase of research, 48 participants (16 African-American, 15 Asian/Pacific Islanders, 12 Latina, and 5 other ethnicity with mixed ethnic background) participated in focus groups. In the second phase, 332 participants (112 African-American, 110 Latina, and 110 Asian/Pacific Islanders) completed the structured questionnaire interview.

Procedures

Focus groups: Seven focus groups were held. A pilot focus group consisted of African-American, API, and Latina participants, followed by six ethnic-specific groups for African-American, API, or Latina participants (two focus groups in each ethnicity). A Spanish-bilingual MtF facilitator led the discussion using a semi-structured protocol. Focus groups were tape-recorded and transcribed verbatim; those conducted in Spanish were transcribed into Spanish then translated into English. Data were analyzed by a team of researchers using standard ethnographic methods (Strauss and Corbin, 1998) including thematic coding and memo-writing (see Nemoto et al., 2004a, in detail).

Individual survey interviews: Participants were interviewed by one of three MtF transgender outreach workers, matched according to ethnicity. The survey was translated into Spanish and then translated back into English to ensure comparability; approximately half of the Latinas were interviewed in Spanish. All other participants were interviewed in English.

Of the measures relevant to this article, we asked participants about (a) demographic characteristics such as age, gender identity, sexual orientation, income, and education; (b) general health and social services needed during the past year; (c) general health and social services received during the past year; (d) gender transition procedures conducted; (e) where they conducted their gender transition procedures; and (f) perceptions of barriers to health and social services. The measures of the questionnaire used either anchored questions (e.g., demographics) or Likert-type scales (e.g., "I don't go to the doctor because they're insensitive to transgender issues" rated from *1 = Strongly Disagree* to *5 = Strongly Agree*). Additional measures included the Center for Epidemiological Scale for Depression (Radloff, 1977); the Rosenberg Self-Esteem scale (Rosenberg, 1965); AIDS knowledge (Nemoto et al., 1999); transphobia (i.e., experiences of discrimination due to their transgender identity, modified from a homophobia scale by Diaz, Ayala, Bein, Henne, & Marin, 2001); self-efficacy to use condoms with private sex partners (Nemoto et al., 2004b); and economic pressure (Nemoto et al., 2004b). We also asked about various HIV risk behaviors including whether participants had ever engaged in unprotected receptive anal sex with private partners during the past 30 days.

Statistical Analysis

All analyses were performed using SPSS, Standard Version, Release 10.0.5. Frequencies were used to summarize health behaviors and demographic characteristics. One-way ANOVAs and Chi-square tests were used to examine differences across ethnic groups and, if significant group differences emerged, bivariate logistic regressions provided odds ratios (OR) and 95% confidence intervals (CI) between groups. In most cases, the lowest-frequency group was selected as the reference group (RG) for computing odds ratios logistic regressions. Pearson correlation coefficients were used to examine the associations between barriers to utilizing services and psychosocial, AIDS knowledge, or behavioral measures.

RESULTS

Focus Group Findings

Participants' comments indicated the scarcity of health and social service programs for the MtF transgender community in San Francisco. Through coding and thematic analysis of focus group data, we found persistent dissatisfaction with existing service programs for this community. Discontent with health and social services derived from four general factors: (1) inadequate programs for transgender clients, (2) inadequate spaces and facilities for transgender clients, (3) staff's insensitivity toward transgender issues and individuals, (4) prejudice expressed by other clients.

The first two factors were closely related and pointed to a need for transgender-specific health services. Commenting on a range of services, from drug treatment to public health clinics to homeless shelters, participants stated that many agencies in San Francisco lacked a fundamental understanding of transgenderism and transgender identity and consequently, could not address the specific needs of these clients. Several programs lacked basic information, resources, and protocols for addressing transgender health, such as how to accommodate hormone use among transgender persons in substance abuse treatment, how to support individuals in the process of gender transition, and how to educate providers about the procedures and risks associated with hormones and surgeries. Service programs lacked basic guidelines for transgender persons' use of restroom and shower facilities, bed and sleeping arrangements, and transgender-appropriate intake forms and questionnaires.

Frequent references to biased and insensitive staff and clients suggested a lack of appropriate training on transgender life experience, identity, and health needs. For example, one participant expressed a comment shared by many, "I have been to many doctors around the country, and they never know. They would say, 'Well, we never had any transsexuals. What do we do?' So we have to tell the doctors what we wanted." Inadequate information, resources, protocols, and training were viewed by participants as discrimination against transgender persons and barriers to access to health care. A statement by one participant summarizes this point: "In order for us to get help, we need someplace where we're being treated equally. Because when I go somewhere and I don't feel like I'm being treated equally, I'll just leave. It's gonna defeat the whole purpose. If they don't care if I get well, why should I?"

Another issue evinced the need for more sophisticated provider education on hormone use and gender transition processes. For example, many participants described purchasing hormones from underground sources, often imported from Mexico and administered without informed knowledge of side-effects. This may be attributable to the reluctance among service providers in San Francisco to disseminate liquid hormones, allowing only for the prescription of hormone pills. Yet, many transgender persons believe that liquid hormones provide faster and more effective results. One focus group participant reflected on this San Francisco policy, "They don't give out injections, and that forces a lot of the transwomen to go on the streets and get hormones. If I went to L.A., I would be able to go to a clinic where I can receive my hormone shots for free." Consequently, transgender women in San Francisco risk using contaminated liquid hormones purchased from street or underground sources, as well as over-using hormones and silicone due to lack of medical supervision. Several focus group participants reported side effects from inappropriate hormone use, ranging from liver and kidney damage to skin infections and abscesses from unsafe needle use. This appears to be an important issue in the Latina transgender community who most frequently reported the use of hormone and silicone injections. Indeed, some Latina focus group participants described injecting cooking and automobile oils and other solvents to obtain more feminizing effects in their body appearance.

Survey Interview Findings

Participant characteristics: Sociodemographic characteristics of the sample are described elsewhere (Nemoto et al., 2004b). The average age was 34 years (range = 18 to 60 years). More than half (58%) were foreign-born. Over one-third (37%) had less than a high school education, and 53% earned less than $1,000 in the past 30 days. Less than half (48%) had permanent housing. The majority (64%) was single. The three most common self-identified genders were female (36%), pre-operative transgender (31%), and pre-operative transsexual (21%). A majority identified their sexual orientation as heterosexual (85%).

General health services: Participants stated whether they ever needed a number of general health services (Table 1) and social services (Table 2) during the past year. If they reported needing the service, participants also stated whether they received the service.

As shown in Table 1, 59% of the overall sample reported needing STD screening, 46% needed psychological counseling, 41% needed general medical care, 25% needed alternative health care, 22% needed emergency room care, 21% needed treatment for substance use, and 19% reported needing urgent care. Table 1 shows Chi-square test results examining the associations between ethnic groups and needs for each health service and odds ratios for ethnic group comparisons. Asian/Pacific Islanders reported the lowest need for each health service, whereas African-Americans and Latinas reported higher health service needs than Asian/Pacific Islanders.

Table 1 also shows frequencies of service received and results of Chi-square tests. Participants reported fairly high levels of having received most health services. Substance use

TABLE 1. Health Services Needed and Received During the Past Year by Ethnicity

Type of Service	Needed[1]	Chi-square[3]	OR (95% CI)	Received[2]	Chi-square[3]
General medical	41%	74.18**		99%	2.06
African-American	70%		15.73 (7.89-31.38)	100%	
Latina	41%		4.74 (2.41-9.35)	98%	
Asian/Pacific Islander	13%		Reference group	100%	
Urgent care	19%	19.07**		99%	2.69
African-American	32%		4.55 (2.12-9.75)	100%	
Latina	16%		1.83 (.80-4.19)	94%	
Asian/Pacific Islander	9%		Reference group	100%	
Substance treatment	21%	32.65**		79%	1.00
African-American	38%		6.99 (3.20-15.27)	79%	
Latina	16%		2.20 (.94-5.13)	83%	
Asian/Pacific Islander	8%		Reference group	67%	
Counseling	46%	10.71**		88%	3.56
African-American	58%		2.42 (1.41-4.15)	83%	
Latina	45%		1.41 (.81-2.41)	90%	
Asian/Pacific Islander	36%		Reference group	95%	
STD screening	59%	13.77**		98%	1.72
African-American	58%		1.54 (.91-2.62)	95%	
Latina	72%		2.84 (1.63-4.97)	99%	
Asian/Pacific Islander	47%		Reference group	98%	
Emergency room	22%	14.05**		97%	3.23
African-American	25%		3.00 (1.41-6.39)	93%	
Latina	30%		3.86 (1.83-8.12)	100%	
Asian/Pacific Islander	10%		Reference group	100%	
Alternative care	25%	26.91**		94%	7.82
African-American	30%		4.89 (2.22-10.80)	85%	
Latina	37%		6.67 (3.04-14.60)	100%	
Asian/Pacific Islander	8%		Reference group	100%	

Notes: [1]Denominators: 332 for overall sample; 112 for African-Americans; 110 for Latinas; 110 for Asian/Pacific Islanders
[2]Denominators: Sub-sample of participants who needed the service
[3]No asterisks (no significant ethnic difference)
**$p < .01$

treatment proved to be an exception, however, with only 79% of those who reported a need for treatment stating that they received treatment. No significant ethnic differences emerged in receiving health care.

As shown in Table 2, the most common social services needed during the past year were spiritual support (39%), followed by food services (36%), general assistance (35%), housing (33%), job training (22%), and job placement (21%). There were significant ethnic differences in need for social services. Asian/Pacific Islanders generally reported the least need whereas African-Americans and Latinas reported higher social service needs.

Table 2 also shows percentages of individuals who reported needs for social services and received specific services, as well as Chi-square test results. High levels of receiving needed services were reported for spiritual support

TABLE 2. Social Services Needed and Received During the Past Year by Ethnicity

Type of Service	Needed[1]	Chi-square	OR (95% CI)	Received[2]	Chi-square	OR (95% CI)
Housing	33%	36.18**		57%	5.43	---
African-American	46%		6.83 (3.37-13.82)	49%		---
Latina	42%		5.87 (2.89-11.93)	70%		---
Asian/Pacific Islander	11%		Reference group	42%		
Food	36%	27.08**		85%	2.99	
African-American	49%		4.62 (2.49-8.57)	91%		---
Latina	43%		3.57 (1.92-6.66)	79%		---
Asian/Pacific Islander	17%		Reference group	84%		---
Job training	22%	10.42**		57%	7.33*	
African-American	32%		2.78 (1.43-5.39)	42%		.21 (.06 -.70)
Latina	20%		1.46 (.72-2.98)	77%		Reference group
Asian/Pacific Islander	15%		Reference group	63%		.49 (.12-2.03)
General assistance	35%	56.56**		83%	4.71	
African-American	61%		9.78 (5.04-18.99)	87%		---
Latina	29%		2.59 (1.31-5.14)	72%		---
Asian/Pacific Islander	14%		Reference group	83%		---
Spiritual support	39%	44.83**		93%	2.34	
African-American	62%		7.22 (3.90-13.37)	90%		---
Latina	36%		2.47 (1.33-4.61)	97%		---
Asian/Pacific Islander	18%		Reference group	95%		---
Utility payment	11%	4.87		71%	3.14	
African-American	14%		---	81%		---
Latina	12%		---	53%		---
Asian/Pacific Islander	6%		---	83%		---
Temporary shelter	19%	25.76**		87%	2.57	
African-American	29%		10.60 (3.60-31.19)	94%		---
Latina	25%		8.62 (2.90-25.60)	82%		---
Asian/Pacific Islander	4%		Reference group	75%		---
Job placement	21%	18.92**		74%	1.19	
African-American	29%		5.10 (2.23-11.67)	72%		---
Latina	27%		4.78 (2.08-11.00)	80%		---
Asian/Pacific Islander	7%		Reference group	63%		---
Unemployment	11%	3.72		57%	2.92	
African-American	14%		---	50%		---
Latina	11%		---	50%		---
Asian/Pacific Islander	6%		---	86%		---
Rape crisis	5%	6.33*		71%	1.25	
African-American	8%		9.52 (1.19-76.44)	78%		---
Latina	6%		7.40 (.89-61.20)	57%		---
Asian/Pacific Islander	1%		Reference group	100%		---

TABLE 2 (continued)

Type of Service	Needed[1]	Chi-square	OR (95% CI)	Received[2]	Chi-square	OR (95% CI)
Legal aid	16%	9.85**		85%	.33	
African-American	22%		3.47 (1.48-8.13)	88%		---
Latina	20%		3.19 (1.35-7.52)	82%		---
Asian/Pacific Islander	7%		Reference group	88%		---
Crisis intervention	12%	11.39**		87%	2.02	
African-American	18%		5.76 (1.90-17.47)	80%		---
Latina	14%		4.18 (1.34-13.05)	93%		---
Asian/Pacific Islander	4%		Reference group	100%		---

Notes: [1]Denominators: 332 for overall sample; 112 for African-Americans; 110 for Latinas; 110 for Asian/Pacific Islanders
[2]Denominators: Subsample of participants who needed the service
**$p < .01$
*$p < .05$

(93%), temporary shelter (87%), crisis intervention (87%), legal aid (85%), food (85%), and general assistance (83%). However, participants received only moderate levels of housing services (57%), job training (57%), unemployment (57%), utility payment services (71%), rape crisis services (71%), and job placement services (74%). A marginally significant ethnic difference emerged in job training services; that is, African-Americans were less likely to receive job training compared to Latinas.

Gender transition procedures: Participants described a variety of gender transition procedures they had undergone–ranging from using hormones and silicone to various forms of surgery. Table 3 shows frequencies, Chi-square test results, and odds rations between ethnic group comparisons.

Most (91%) of the sample had a history of hormone use and three-quarters of them (75%) were currently using hormones. The majority of the sample also had a history of injecting hormones (67%) and a third of them (32%) were currently injecting hormones. Latinas (80%) were significantly more likely to have ever injected hormones compared to African-Americans (60%) and Asians and Pacific Islanders (60%). Overall, 22% had ever had silicone injections, highest among Latinas (41%) compared to African-Americans (13%) and Asians and Pacific Islanders (12%). Relative to Asian and Pacific Islanders, Latinas were 4 times as likely to have ever injected hormones, and over 5 times more likely to have had silicone injections (see Table 3).

Nearly a third of the sample (30%) had conducted some form of gender-related surgery, highest among Asians and Pacific Islanders (39%) and Latinas (31%). A quarter (25%) of the sample reported having breast implants, and 13% reported having some form of facial plastic surgery. Other surgical procedures included vaginoplasty (9%), testicle removal (10%), hip enlargement (7%), and Adam's apple reduction (6%). Asians and Pacific Islanders were significantly more likely to have had breast implants (34%), vaginoplasty (16%), testicle removal (16%), Adam's apple reduction (10%), and facial surgery (16%), whereas Latinas were most likely to have had hip enlargement procedures (13%).

Over half (59%) of the sample had plans for future types of gender-related surgical procedures. Planned procedures included breast implants (37%), vaginoplasty (35%), testicle removal (32%), hip enlargement (18%), Adam's apple reduction (12%), and facial surgery (27%). African-Americans were most likely to be planning for vaginoplasty (75%), and Latinas were most likely to be planing for hip enlargement (56%), Adam's apple reduction (35%), and facial surgery (76%).

Sources of gender transition procedures: Participants listed all sources that provided them with hormones, performed hormone injections, and performed silicone injections. They also described where they conducted each gender transition procedure.

As Table 4 shows, the majority (74%) reported being prescribed hormones from a doc-

TABLE 3. Gender Transition Procedures[1]

	%	Chi-square	OR (95% CI)
Ever used hormones			
Overall	91%	3.22	
African-American	95%		---
Latina	89%		---
Asian/Pacific Islander	88%		---
Currently using hormones			
Overall	75%	3.63	
African-American	77%		---
Latina	64%		---
Asian/Pacific Islander	62%		---
Ever injected hormones			
Overall	67%	20.32**	
African-American	60%		.78 (.44-1.40)
Latina	80%		4.00 (1.83-8.75)
Asian/Pacific Islander	60%		Reference group
Currently injecting hormones			
Overall	32%	1.21	
African-American	29%		---
Latina	41%		---
Asian/Pacific Islander	25%		Reference group
Ever had silicone injections			
Overall	22%	34.14**	
African-American	13%		1.14 (.52-2.53)
Latina	41%		5.11 (2.56-10.22)
Asian/Pacific Islander	12%		Reference group
Ever had any sex reassignment procedures conducted			
Overall	30%	11.49**	
African-American	19%		Reference group
Latina	31%		1.94 (1.03-3.61)
Asian/Pacific Islander	39%		2.82 (1.53-5.20)
Type of procedures conducted			
Breast implants			
Overall	25%	8.16*	
African-American	17%		Reference group
Latina	26%		1.67 (.87-3.21)
Asian/Pacific Islander	34%		2.48 (1.32-4.67)
Vaginoplasty			
Overall	9%	7.51*	
African-American	5%		Reference group
Latina	7%		1.38 (.46-4.13)
Asian/Pacific Islander	16%		3.22 (1.22-8.52)
Testicle removal			
Overall	10%	6.93*	
African-American	6%		Reference group
Latina	8%		1.34 (.48-3.72)
Asian/Pacific Islander	16%		2.93 (1.17-7.33)

TABLE 3 (continued)

	%	Chi-square	OR (95% CI)
Hip enlargement			
Overall	7%	11.02**	
African-American	5%		3.05 (.60-15.43)
Latina	13%		7.86 (1.74-35.42)
Asian/Pacific Islander	2%		Reference group
Adam's apple reduction			
Overall	6%	5.94*	
African-American	3%		Reference group
Latina	5%		1.73 (.40-7.42)
Asian/Pacific Islander	10%		4.04 (1.09-14.89)
Facial surgery			
Overall	13%	8.69**	
African-American	5%		Reference group
Latina	17%		3.68 (1.41-9.62)
Asian/Pacific Islander	16%		3.45 (1.32-9.06)
Types of procedures planned for the future			
Any sexual reassignment procedure			
Overall	59%	5.94	
African-American	62%		---
Latina	69%		---
Asian/Pacific Islander	53%		---
Breast implants			
Overall	37%	2.20	
African-American	57%		---
Latina	69%		---
Asian/Pacific Islander	63%		---
Vaginoplasty			
Overall	35%	9.01*	
African-American	75%		2.46 (1.14-5.32)
Latina	51%		.86 (.43-1.72)
Asian/Pacific Islander	54%		Reference group
Testicle removal			
Overall	32%	5.34	
African-American	67%		---
Latina	48%		---
Asian/Pacific Islander	51%		---
Hip enlargement			
Overall	18%	42.28**	
African-American	19%		3.12 (.94-10.30)
Latina	56%		16.86 (5.34-51.36)
Asian/Pacific Islander	7%		Reference group
Adam's apple reduction			
Overall	12%	17.37**	
African-American	14%		2.21 (.64-7.61)
Latina	35%		7.03 (2.29-21.59)
Asian/Pacific Islander	7%		Reference group
Facial surgery			
Overall	27%	42.31**	
African-American	30%		1.21 (.54-2.69)
Latina	76%		8.87 (4.01-19.59)
Asian/Pacific Islander	26%		Reference group

Notes: [1]112 African-Americans, 110 Asian/Pacific Islanders, 110 Latinas
**$p < .01$
*$p < .05$

TABLE 4. Source of Gender Transition Procedures[1]

Received hormones from:	%
Doctor's prescription	74%
Hospital or Clinic	33%
Friend	32%
Mexico	21%
Other non-prescription source	9%
Hormones currently injected by:	
Yourself	46%
Friend	40%
Medical professional in the U.S.	29%
Medical professional in another country	2%
Silicone injections performed by:	
Non-medical person, who regularly performs this service for transgender persons	49%
Medical professional in the U.S.	18%
Friend	18%
Medical professional in another country	15%
Yourself	1%
Gender-related surgeries conducted:	
In a U.S. medical setting	67%
In a non-U.S. medical setting	43%
Mexico	22%
Thailand	15%
Canada	1%
France	1%
Brazil	1%
In a U.S. non-medical setting	2%

Note: [1]Denominator includes only those who had engaged in each behavior.

tor, and 33% received hormones from a hospital or clinic. However, 32% reported acquiring hormones from friends, 21% from Mexico (where hormones are sold without prescription), and 9% from another non-prescription source (usually from street vendors). Among participants who currently were injecting hormones, 46% reported injecting themselves, 40% were injected by friends, 29% by medical professionals in the United States, and 2% by medical professionals in another country (not mutually exclusive for these categories).

For participants who reported ever having silicone injections, 49% received injections by a non-medical person–often a vendor who sells silicone and regularly conducts silicone injections for MtF transgender persons in San Francisco. Silicone injections had also been provided by medical professionals in the United States (18%), by friends (18%), and by medical professionals outside of the United States (15%).

Among those who had ever had gender-related surgeries, the majority (67%) were con-

ducted in a United States medical setting. Foreign surgeries were also common (43%), with Mexico (22%) and Thailand (15%) being frequent sites for surgical procedures.

Perceived barriers to health services: Three measures of perceived barriers to health services were included in the survey: perceived barriers to health care for transgender persons, perceived barriers to health care for people of color, and perceived barriers to drug treatment for transgender persons of color. Table 5 lists items for each measure, mean values, and standard deviations. Each measure showed strong internal reliability (alpha = .86 for health care barriers for transgender persons, .93 for health care for people of color, and .95 for drug treatment barriers for transgender persons of color), and the measures intercorrelated significantly (r = .35 to .62, all p values < .01).

We used one-way ANOVAs to test for ethnic group differences on these barrier measures. We found no significant ethnic differences on perceived barriers to health care for transgender persons (Ms: 2.14 for African-

TABLE 5. Perceived Barriers to Health Services

Perceived barriers to health care for transgender persons	Mean (SD)	Percentage Agree/Strongly agree
I don't go to a free transgender clinic because of the long waiting list.	2.63 (1.23)	34%
I don't go to the doctor or a clinic because they're not knowledgeable about transgender issues.	2.32 (1.09)	21%
I don't go to the doctor because they're insensitive to transgender issues.	2.34 (1.08)	22%
I don't go to the doctor because I've had degrading experiences related to being transgender.	2.11 (.96)	13%
I don't know of any affordable transgender clinics.	2.17 (.97)	13%
I avoid transgender clinics because I don't want other transgender persons to see me.	2.03 (.95)	10%
Perceived barriers to health care for people of color		
I don't go to the doctor or a clinic because the staff there don't speak my native language.	1.75 (.76)	5%
It's hard for me to find out information about health services because most of the information is printed in English.	1.78 (.82)	6%
I don't go to the doctor or a clinic because they're not knowledgeable about issues related to my race/ethnicity.	1.92 (.84)	8%
I don't go to the doctor or a clinic because they're insensitive to issues related to my race/ethnicity.	1.94 (.88)	9%
I don't go to the doctor or a hospital because I've had degrading experiences.	1.94 (.89)	9%
Perceived barriers to drug treatment for transgender persons of color		
I wouldn't go to a drug treatment program because they're not knowledgeable about transgender issues.	2.38 (1.04)	15%
I wouldn't go to a drug treatment program because they're insensitive to transgender issues.	2.43 (1.06)	16%
I wouldn't go to a drug treatment program because I've had degrading experiences there related to being transgender.	2.35 (1.02)	13%
I wouldn't go to a drug treatment program because they're not knowledgeable about issues related to my race or ethnicity.	2.24 (.94)	8%
I wouldn't go to a drug treatment program because they're insensitive to issues related to my race or ethnicity.	2.26 (.95)	8%
I wouldn't go to a drug treatment program because I've had degrading experiences there related to my race or ethnicity.	2.24 (.93)	8%

American, 2.31 for Asian and Pacific Islanders, 2.35 for Latinas; p = ns). Significant ethnic differences emerged for the other measures. For perceived barriers to health care for people of color, Latinas had the highest score (M = 2.29) followed by Asian and Pacific Islanders (M = 1.85) and African-Americans with the lowest score (M = 1.64), $F(2, 327) = 26.09, p < .01$. For perceived barriers to drug treatment for transgender persons of color, Latinas again had the highest score (M = 2.62) followed by African-Americans (M = 2.31) and Asian and Pacific Islanders with the lowest score (M = 2.00), $F(2, 278) = 12.56, p < .01$.

Bivariate correlations were conducted to examine the associations between these three perceived barriers toward health services and measures of psychological variables, AIDS knowledge, self-efficacy to use condoms, and frequency of unprotected receptive anal sex. As Table 6 shows, all three measures were significantly correlated with increased depression, lower self-esteem, increased transphobia, increased economic pressure, lower AIDS-knowledge, lower self-efficacy to use condoms with private partners, and increased number of times engaging in unprotected receptive anal sex with private partners during the past month (all p values < .01, except one correlation between barriers to drug treatment and frequency of the sexual risk behavior).

DISCUSSION

In this article, we sought to identify health care needs, service utilization rates, and perceptions of barriers toward utilizing services among MtF transgender persons in San Francisco. Our survey findings indicated strong needs for a range of health and social services in this community. Although participants reported relatively moderate to high rates of health service utilization, social service utilization levels tended to be lower than medical utilization rates. Moreover, findings from focus groups revealed that, despite adequate levels of receiving many needed services, members of the MtF transgender community were generally dissatisfied with the quality of health and social services currently provided. Previous studies also reported MtF transgender persons dissatisfaction with quality of services provided at health and social service agencies (Bockting et al., 1998; Clements et al., 1999). Quantitative findings indicated that perceived barriers against utilizing heath care for transgender persons and for people of color were strongly and positively correlated with the frequency of engaging in risky sexual behaviors (unprotected receptive anal sex with private partners), lower levels of AIDS knowledge and self-efficacy to practice safe sex, and psychological problems (depression, low self-esteem, transphobic experience, and economic pressure). These results clearly indicate that ethnic minority MtF transgender persons who experience negative interactions with health providers and face discrimination in the health care system feel strong barriers to utilizing health care services, and consequently exacerbate health disparities (Clements et al., 1999; Kenagy, 2005). Transphobia experience, depression, and economic pressure would also contribute to the barriers to utilizing services experienced by MtF transgender persons of color. This vicious cycle must be eliminated by developing health intervention programs specific to MtF transgender persons.

A large portion of the sample reported needs for basic health services during the past year including general medical care, counseling, and STD screening, as well as social services including housing, food, general assistance, and spiritual support. Gender transition-related services were particularly needed, as three-quarters of the sample reported current hormone use, one-third reported currently injecting hormones, and over half reported planning for some form of gender-related surgery in the future such as breast implants and vaginoplasty.

Although we did not include white MtF transgender persons in our study samples, ethnic disparities were found for almost every health and social service needed, as well as for most gender transition-related procedures. African-American MtF transgender persons reported particularly high levels of need for general medical services, substance use treatment, psychological counseling, STD screening, housing services, food assistance, job training, general assistance/SSI, and spiritual support. Latina MtF transgender persons reported particularly high levels of need for general medical services, psychological counseling, STD screening, alternative care, health services, food assistance, and spiritual support. Asian and Pacific Islander MtF transgender persons reported high levels of need for psychological counseling and STD screening. Although all ethnic groups reported engaging in gender-confirmation surgery or therapy such as hormone therapy and breast implants, and planning for future surgeries, Latinas reported the highest rates of injecting hormones and silicone, planning for hip enlargement (ostensibly through silicone implants, silicone injections, or injecting oils), Adam's apple reduction, and facial surgery. Similarly, African-Americans reported the highest rates of planning for future vaginoplasty. Asian and Pacific Islanders, in contrast, were most likely to have had sex reassignment surgery such as breast implants, vaginoplasty, testicle removal, and Adam's apple reduction.

Rates of service utilization varied depending on the type of service. For most health services, the overall levels of receiving care were generally in the ninetieth percentile. Substance abuse treatment and psychological counseling proved to be exceptions, with participants reporting lower utilization levels for both. Likewise, levels of receiving social services such as housing, job training, job placement, unemployment, and rape crisis were markedly lower than for health services.

Barrier measures showed ethnic disparities in perceptions of health barriers for transgender persons of color. Latina transgender persons reported the highest rates of perceived barriers to health care for people of color and barriers to drug treatment for transgender persons of color. Perceived barriers to health ser-

TABLE 6. Correlation Coefficient Between Perceived Barriers to Health Services and Psychological Variables, AIDS Knowledge, Self-Efficacy, or Unprotected Sex

	Form of health care barrier		
	Health care for transgender persons	Health care for people of color	Drug treatment for transgender persons of color
Depression	.17**	.35**	.30**
Self-esteem	−.21**	−.38**	.30**
Transphobia	.14**	.28**	.38**
Economic pressure	.33**	.40**	.32**
AIDS knowledge	−.16**	−.36**	−.22**
Self-efficacy to use condoms with private partners	−.20**	−.32**	−.26**
Number of times had unprotected receptive anal sex with private partners	.22**	.32**	.08

Notes: **$p < .01$

vices were significantly associated with increased depression, transphobia, economic pressure, and lower self-esteem, as well as with health risks such as lower self-efficacy to use condoms with private partners and increase unprotected receptive anal sex with private partners. This suggests that barriers toward health care form an important part of the psychosocial context of HIV risk among MtF transgender persons in San Francisco. Another study (Nemoto et al., 2004b) indicated that compared with Asian and Pacific Islander MtF transgender persons, Latina MtF transgender persons had significantly higher levels of psychological problems and that African-American MtF transgender persons had engaged in higher levels of sexual risk behaviors. It is possible that low levels of utilization of medical and social services and perceived strong barriers toward utilizing services among Latina and African-American MtF transgender persons have contributed to their psychological problems and high risk behaviors for HIV infection.

There are important limitations to these findings. First, our sample included only MtF transgender persons of color who identify as AfricanAmerican, Asian and Pacific Islander, or Latina; those who identify as white/Caucasian, Native American, or other were not eligible to participate. It is possible that the health issues for other MtF transgender racial/ethnic groups are markedly different. Second, our recruitment procedure used convenient sampling methods and referrals from service providers and from participants in the study, so we may not have a representative sample of MtF transgender persons of color in San Francisco. Finally, our methods relied on self-report of highly personal information, so self-presentation concerns and limited recall may have biased some findings.

The findings presented here offer important perspectives on the state of health and social services for MtF transgender persons of color. San Francisco is one of the metropolitan areas in the U.S. with a distinguished reputation for acknowledging and addressing the needs of sexual and gender minorities. Yet the current situation for the MtF transgender community appears less than ideal. MtF transgender persons reported high levels of service utilization for meeting their basic general health needs, but less adequate rates of service utilization for an array of social services, substance abuse treatment, psychological counseling, and gender confirmation surgery and treatment services such as hormone therapy. Perceived barriers to health care were associated with poor psychosocial functioning as well as increased HIV risk. Dissatisfaction with health and social service providers appeared to be associated with lack of transgender-appropriate programs and resources, inadequate sensitivity training of staff and clients regarding transgenderism. Few transgender-specific services address gender transition procedures and the psychosocial vulnerabilities to HIV, drug use, and mental health problems. Findings also pointed to strengths among health and social services for MtF transgender persons in San

Francisco. For example, several focus group participants praised the efforts of some community-based organizations for their programs targeting the MtF transgender community. Coalitions between staff from these agencies, researchers, and community members are necessary to push the boundaries of public health and increase the range and quality of services for San Francisco's MtF transgender community.

REFERENCES

Bockting, W. O. (1997) The assessment and treatment of gender dysphoria. *Directions in Clinical Counseling Psychology*, 7: 1-23.

Bockting, W. O., Robinson, B. E., and Rosser, B. R. S. (1998) Transgender HIV prevention: A qualitative needs assessment. *AIDS Care*, 10: 505-526.

Clements, K., Wilkinson, W., Kitano, K., and Marx, R. (1999). HIV prevention and health service needs of the transgender community in San Francisco. *The International Journal of Transgenderism, 3*, 1 & 2, http://www.symposion.com/ijt/hiv_risk/clements.htm.

Clements-Nolle, K., Marx, R., Guzman, R., and Katz, M. (2001) HIV prevalence, risk behaviors, health care use, and mental health status of transgender persons: Implications for public health intervention. *American Journal of Public Health*, 91: 915-921.

Cole, S. S., Denny, D., Eyler, A. E., and Samons, S. L. (2000) Issues of transgender. In L. T. Szuchman and F. Muscarella, (Eds.), 149-195. *Psychological perspectives on human sexuality*. New York: John Wiley and Sons, Inc.

Diaz, R. M. (1998) *Latino gay men and HIV: Culture, sexuality, and risk behavior*. New York: Routledge.

Diaz, R. M., Ayala, G., Bein, E., Henne, J., and Marin, B. V. (2001). The impact of homophobia, poverty, and racism on the mental health of gay and bisexual Latino men: Findings from 3 US cities. *American Journal of Public Health*, 91: 927-932.

Elifson, K. W., Boles, J., Posey, E., Sweat, M., Darrow, W., and Elsea, W. (1993) Male transvestite prostitutes and HIV risk. *American Journal of Public Health*, 83: 260-262.

Gagne, P., Tewksbury, R., and McGaughey, D. (1997) Coming out and crossing over: Identity formation and proclamation in a transgender community. *Gender and Society*, 11: 478-508.

Kenagy, G. P. (2005). Transgender health: Findings from two needs assessment studies in Philadelphia. *Health and Social Work, 30(1)*, 19-26.

Kreiss, J. L. and Patterson, D. L. (1997) Psychosocial issues in primary care of lesbian, gay, and bisexual and transgender youth. *Journal of Pediatric Health Care*, 11: 266-274.

Lombardi, E. L. (2001) Enhancing transgender care. *American Journal of Public Health*, 91: 869-872.

Nemoto, T., Luke, D., Mamo, L., Ching, A., and Patria, J. (1999) HIV risk behaviors among male-to-female transgenders in comparison with homosexual or bisexual females. *AIDS Care*, 11: 297-312.

Nemoto, T., Operario, D., Keatley, J., and Villegas, D. (2004a) Social context of HIV risk behaviours among male-to-female transgenders of colour. *AIDS CARE, 16(6)*, 724-735.

Nemoto, T., Operario, D., Keatley, J., Han, L., and Soma, T. (2004b) HIV risk behaviors among male-to-female transgender persons of color in San Francisco. *American Journal of Public Health*, 94: 1193-1199.

Nemoto, T., Operario, D., Keatley, J., Nguyen, H., and Sugano, E. (2005) Promoting health for transgender women: Transgender Resources and Neighborhood Space (TRANS) Program in San Francisco. *American Journal of Public Health*, 382-384.

Radloff, L. S. (1977) The CES-D scale: A self-report depression scale for research in the general population. *Applied Psychological Measurement*, 1: 385-401.

Rosenberg, M. (1965) *Society and the Adolescent Self-image*. Princeton: Princeton University Press.

San Francisco Department of Public Health. (1998) *San Francisco HIV Epidemiology Report*. San Francisco: SFDPH.

San Francisco Department of Public Health. (1999) *The transgender community health project: Descriptive results*. San Francisco: SFDPH.

Springer, E. A. (1999) *Effective HIV prevention with marginalized populations: The harm reduction model of behavior change*. Paper presented at the National HIV Prevention Conference, Atlanta.

Strauss, A., and Corbin, J. (1998). *Basics of qualitative research: Techniques and procedures for developing grounded theory* (2nd ed.). Thousand Oaks, CA: Sage Publications.

Verschoor, A. M., and Poortinga, J. (1988) Psychosocial differences between Dutch male and female transsexuals. *Archives of Sexual Behavior*, 17: 173-178.

Zevin, B. (2000) Demographics of the transgender clinic at San Francisco's Tom Waddell Center. Paper presented at the University of California San Francisco Transgender Care Conference, San Francisco.

The Role of Male Sexual Partners in HIV Infection Among Male-to-Female Transgendered Individuals

Dara L. Coan, MPH
Willow Schrager, MPP
Tracey Packer, MPH

SUMMARY. Male-to-female transgendered persons (MtF) in San Francisco have very high HIV prevalence and incidence. To explore possible sources for these high rates of HIV infection, a rapid needs assessment was conducted using two methods: (1) an interviewer-administered, mostly closed-ended survey with the male partners of MtF persons, and (2) focus groups with MtF persons. Five main themes were evident from the findings: (1) male partners of MtF persons are of all ages, races, sexual orientations, and socioeconomic backgrounds; (2) high-risk sex occurs between MtF persons and their male sexual partners, despite a high level of concern about HIV among both the male and MtF study participants; (3) drug use appears to play a role in unsafe sex between MtF and their male partners; (4) male partners of MtF persons may represent a possible bridge for HIV transmission among different populations, given that they reported sex with male and female partners, as well as transgendered partners; and (5) men engaging in receptive anal sex with MtF partners probably occurs more frequently than reported by the male participants, given the comments of MtF study participants. The results indicate a need for creative, community-based HIV prevention strategies that target the male partners of MtF transgendered persons. *[Article copies available for a fee from The Haworth Document Delivery Service: 1-800-HAWORTH. E-mail address: <docdelivery@ haworthpress.com> Website: <http://www.HaworthPress.com> © 2005 by The Haworth Press, Inc. All rights reserved.]*

KEYWORDS. Transgender, sexual partners, male-to-female, HIV/AIDS

Dara L. Coan, MPH, was affiliated with Harper+Company Community Research at the time this article was written. She is now affiliated with Community Health Consulting, Berkeley, CA (E-mail: dara@chconsulting.org). Willow Schrager, MPP, was affiliated with Harper+Company Community Research at the time this article was written. She is now affiliated with Bay Area Economics, Berkeley, CA. Tracey Parker, MPH, is affiliated with the San Francisco Department of Public Health.

Please address correspondence to Dara Coan.

The authors thank the HIV Prevention Planning Council for supporting this research, particularly the members of the Strategic Evaluation Committee who developed the idea for this needs assessment. They also thank Willi McFarland and Valerie Rose of the San Francisco Department of Public Health AIDS Office for their assistance with this work. Finally, the authors wish to express their sincere gratitude to Carla Clynes and the other community experts who helped them gain access to this population, without whom this study would not have been possible.

This needs assessment was funded by the San Francisco Department of Public Health, HIV Prevention Section.

[Haworth co-indexing entry note]: "The Role of Male Sexual Partners in HIV Infection Among Male-to-Female Transgendered Individuals." Coan, Dara L., Willow Schrager, and Tracey Packer. Co-published simultaneously in *International Journal of Transgenderism* (The Haworth Medical Press, an imprint of The Haworth Press, Inc.) Vol. 8, No. 2/3, 2005, pp. 21-30; and: *Transgender Health and HIV Prevention: Needs Assessment Studies from Transgender Communities Across the United States* (ed: Walter Bockting, and Eric Avery) The Haworth Medical Press, an imprint of The Haworth Press, Inc., 2005, pp. 21-30. Single or multiple copies of this article are available for a fee from The Haworth Document Delivery Service [1-800-HAWORTH, 9:00 a.m. - 5:00 p.m. (EST). E-mail address: docdelivery@haworthpress.com].

Available online at http://www.haworthpress.com/web/IJT
doi:10.1300/J485v08n02_03

INTRODUCTION

An increasing number of studies in recent years, particularly in San Francisco, have explored HIV risk behaviors and their social context among transgendered individuals. The size of the male-to-female (MtF) transgendered population in San Francisco has been estimated at 3,000,[1] and HIV prevalence and incidence are very high among this group. In a 1997 seroprevalence and risk behavior study, prevalence among MtF was 35%.[2] According to a study using counseling and testing data from July 1997 through June 2000 among repeat transgendered testers, incidence was 7.8 per 100 person-years;[3] in other words, 7.8% of the uninfected population will acquire HIV in any given year. African American MtF are disproportionately affected with an HIV prevalence of 63%, more that twice that for any other racial/ethnic group.[2] African American race/ethnicity was also an independent predictor of HIV seroconversion in the counseling and testing study.[3]

The social, environmental, and psychological factors that lead to these high rates of HIV infection among MtF include poverty, drug use, commercial sex work performed out of economic necessity, low self-esteem, and discrimination (in general, and by health and social service providers), among other issues.[1] The San Francisco Department of Public Health funds several community-based HIV prevention agencies to provide services to the transgender population to address some of these issues, as well as to encourage and provide HIV testing and promote HIV risk reduction.

One question that has not been fully answered is: What are the sources of new infections among MtF persons? One possible source is their male sexual partners. Is HIV infection among the male partners contributing to new HIV infections among MtF persons? Are the male partners at risk of acquiring HIV from their MtF or other partners? Do HIV-positive men engage in high-risk sex with MtF persons? To explore these and other questions, a rapid assessment focusing on the male partners of MtF persons was proposed by the HIV Prevention Planning Council, a community advisory board that works with the HIV Prevention Section of the Department of Public Health. The rapid assessment methodology was chosen for its capacity to collect and report on data in a short period of time, which was necessary to provide the community advisory board with information it could use to make recommendations regarding resources and services for this population. This methodology combines scientific rigor with a community-based approach and serves as a preliminary inquiry into issues of concern, with the goal of identifying recommendations for prevention and areas for future study. To our knowledge, this study is the first to explore HIV transmission and prevention issues among the male sexual partners of MtF in the United States.

The male sexual partners of MtF include the husbands, boyfriends, casual partners, and sex work clients of MtF. Specific knowledge about this population is limited to that provided by a handful of studies in which MtF individuals (most of whom have not had sexual reassignment surgery/vaginoplasty) reported information about their male sexual partners. Studies report the following findings and conclusions:

- Male sexual partners of MtF are of all sexual orientations–heterosexual, bisexual, and homosexual[4]–but usually heterosexual or bisexual.[5,6] The clients of MtF sex workers are most frequently heterosexual.[7]
- Men engage in both anal insertive and receptive intercourse with their MtF partners, although insertive intercourse is more common.[4,8,9]
- Both insertive and receptive oral sex were found to be common, with the men being the insertive partners more often than the MtF transgendered persons.[4]
- Male sexual partners of MtF are stigmatized for their attraction to transgendered persons and are considered deviant, thus increasing the likelihood of secretive relationships and sexual encounters.[7,10]
- Male partners of MtF have the greatest power in the sexual relationship, because affirmation of identity and social status among peers for a transgendered person often depends on having relationship(s) or sexual encounter(s) with a man, thus creating a power imbalance.[7,10]

- In general, men who have romantic or primary relationships with transgendered persons are not connected to prevention or other community support networks. Those who are connected to the service system do not feel that existing HIV prevention education meets their needs.[6]
- Men who are clients of transgendered sex workers, and who are often married men, actively pursue unsafe sex practices, using offers of increased financial compensation for performing unsafe sex. These men are very difficult to reach with prevention messages.[6]

The common limitation among these prior studies for understanding sexual risk behaviors among the male partners of MtF persons is that the subjects were all transgendered persons; thus, any information about the male partners was gleaned from data provided by the transgendered study participants and not the men themselves. This needs assessment adds to the information provided by previous studies because it incorporates not only the perspective of MtF persons, but also the direct reports of their male partners.

METHODS

Interviews with Male Sexual Partners of MtF Transgendered

Participants

In February/March 2001, a nonrandom (convenience and snowball) sample of men who have sex with MtF persons was recruited from bars and other street and community locations in San Francisco where MtF persons and their male partners are known to congregate. In addition, the study interviewers and other key informants assisted with recruitment by identifying potential respondents in their social networks (e.g., friends, acquaintances, family). To protect anonymity, the key informants asked potential participants to contact us if they were interested.

Fifty-eight men completed the interview, of which 43 (74%) were eligible.[11] The demographics of the sample are shown in Table 1.

TABLE 1. Demographics of Male Partners of MtF Transgendered Persons

Demographic Characteristic	Number (% of sample)
Race/Ethnicity	
African American	10 (23%)
Asian/Pacific Islander	1 (2%)
Latino/Hispanic	20 (47%)
Native American	0 (0%)
White	7 (16%)
Reported more than one race/ethnicity	5 (12%)
Age	
18-29	16 (37%)
30-39	17 (40%)
40-49	9 (21%)
50+	1 (2%)
Sexual Orientation	
Heterosexual/straight	19 (44%)
Bisexual	19 (44%)
Homosexual/gay	3 (7%)
Other*	2 (5%)
Marital Status	
Not married	32 (74%)
Married	8 (19%)
Other (separated, divorced, widowed)	3 (7%)
Self-Reported HIV Status	
HIV-positive	8 (19%)
HIV-negative	19 (44%)
Unknown	2 (5%)
Declined to answer	1 (2%)

*One individual who responded "other" stated that he identified as bisexual and gay, and the other was unable to define his sexual orientation and said "I like transvestites."
Note: Percentages that do not add up to 100% indicate missing data.

All respondents were biological, non-transgendered males. The sample was multiethnic (predominantly Latino and African American), and most respondents were in their twenties and thirties (77%), either heterosexual (44%) or bisexual (44%), and unmarried (74%). Eight individuals (19%) reported being HIV-positive. Two of the eight HIV-positive individuals (25%) identified as heterosexual.

Instruments

The interview protocol consisted of open- and closed-ended questions. First, the interviewer asked a series of questions regarding demographics, including race, age, sexual orientation, and marital status. The interviewer then asked about participants' level of concern regarding HIV/AIDS, followed by questions designed to explore what types of HIV prevention services they would use (e.g., services provided by an agency serving gay and bisexual men, services provided by a doctor). The next set of questions elicited HIV testing history (e.g., when were they last tested) and serostatus.

The longest section of the interview consisted of questions about sexual behaviors with male, female, and transgendered partners. The interview questions in this section distinguished between main or primary partners, casual partners, and commercial sex work partners (i.e., partners with whom there was an exchange of money or drugs for sex). Specifically, participants were asked whether they had various types of sex in the prior six months with each type of partner and how frequently they used condoms for each of the following types of sex: insertive oral sex, receptive oral sex, insertive anal sex, receptive anal sex, and vaginal insertive sex. Unprotected sex was measured using a five-point Likert scale, where participants were asked to consider all the sex they had in the prior six months and to rate whether they used condoms always, most of the time, sometimes, rarely, or never. "Unprotected sex" was defined as any response except "always."

The interview continued with questions about drug and alcohol use, including questions about non-injection (e.g., marijuana) and injection (e.g., heroin) drug use in the prior three months, as well as whether they had injected with previously used needles in the prior three months. At the close of the interview, participants were asked their opinions about how to conduct effective HIV prevention with the male partners of MtF persons.

Procedure

A team of interviewers with prior outreach experience or a history of working with the transgender community were hired and trained to administer a 30- to 45-minute interview. This methodology was chosen as opposed to focus groups because it allows for more privacy and anonymity, which is especially important given the sensitive nature of the questions. Interviews were conducted in both English and Spanish, depending on the respondent's preference. Participants signed an

informed consent before beginning the interview, and twenty-five dollars in cash was offered as an incentive for participation.

Analysis

Quantitative data from the interview were analyzed using SPSS.[12] Analysis consisted of basic descriptive statistics, including frequencies and crosstabulations. Qualitative data from the open-ended interview questions were analyzed using content analysis, whereby themes were identified and described.

Focus Groups with MtF Transgendered Persons

To supplement the interview data, two focus groups were conducted with MtF transgendered persons in March 2001, asking them about their male partners. This methodology was chosen because individuals may underreport certain sexual behaviors that are perceived to carry a stigma (e.g., receptive anal sex). By including the transgender perspective, we aimed to further explore the prevalence and nature of such sexual behaviors.

Participants

Participants for the two focus groups were recruited through flyers posted at approximately 10 local service agencies. The first focus group was held in the Tenderloin area of the city, a low-income and very diverse neighborhood, and consisted of twelve participants. The second group was held just outside the heart of the Tenderloin and consisted of fifteen participants, for a total of twenty-seven participants overall. Participants were diverse in terms of race/ethnicity.

Description of the Participants

There were slight differences in the demographics of participants in the two focus groups held with MtF transgendered individuals. Participants in the first focus group included a greater number of sex workers, reported lower economic status, were predominantly African American, and were more vocal about personal drug use, especially crack cocaine. Many in the second focus group also received payment for sex, but were more likely to have long-term boyfriends, reported higher economic status, were predominantly Asian and Pacific Islander, and included a greater number of post-operative MtF. Despite these differences, findings from the two groups were similar overall. Key findings from both focus groups are therefore presented together.

Instruments

The initial questions on the focus group protocol focused on describing the husbands and boyfriends of MtF persons (e.g., race/ethnicity, sexual orientation, socioeconomic status, types of sex they engage in). The same series of questions were then asked about the male casual partners of MtF persons, as well as the clients of MtF sex workers. Subsequently, the facilitator explored the participants' perceptions of their male partners' level of concern about HIV and how their male partners felt about using condoms during sex. Next, the groups discussed their concerns about men contributing to new HIV infections among MtF persons via sex. Finally, the facilitator sought input from the groups regarding how best to deliver HIV prevention services and messages to their male partners.

Procedure

Focus group discussions lasted approximately 75 minutes and were led by trained facilitators. Due to the sensitive nature of the topics discussed, it was decided that audiotaping might inhibit individuals from participating fully. Therefore, an experienced note-taker took detailed notes at each focus group. Verbal consent was obtained from participants at the beginning of the session, and twenty-five dollars in cash was offered as an incentive for participation.

Analysis

Focus group notes were analyzed using content analysis, in which themes were identified and described. Differences between the two focus groups are noted where appropriate.

RESULTS

Results from Interviews with Male Partners of MtF Transgendered Persons

Sexual Partners of Men Who Have Sex with Transgendered Persons

Only one-fourth (23%) of the sample reported having had sex with only MtF partners in the last six months (Table 2). About half the sample (51%) also had male or female partners (14% had male and 37% had female partners). The remaining fourth (23%) had both male and female partners in addition to their MtF partners. These data suggest possible "bridges" for HIV transmission among MtF persons, their male partners, and other men and women in their sexual networks, if high-risk behavior and HIV prevalence are present. Five of the 19 men (26%) who identified as heterosexual reported having had one or more male (non-transgendered) partners in the last six months, in addition to their MtF partners, reinforcing the notion that sexual identity does not always correlate with behavior. Finally, 81% (n = 35) of the total sample and 75% (n = 6 of 8) of the HIV-positive respondents reported having more than one sexual partner in the last six months.

Sexual Behaviors and Condom Use

Data regarding the sex that respondents had in the prior six months with males, females, and MtF persons are presented in Table 3. Overall, 44% of the respondents (n = 19) reported unprotected anal sex (receptive and/or insertive) with MtF partners. Only 16% (n = 7) reported receptive anal sex, but four of the seven (57%) reported unprotected receptive anal sex with MtF persons. Two men reported having unpro-

TABLE 2. Reported Sexual Partners of Male Partners of MtF Transgendered Persons

Gender of Sexual Partners in Last Six Months	Number (%)
Transgendered partners only	10 (23%)
Transgendered and male partners	6 (14%)
Transgendered and female partners	16 (37%)
Transgendered, male, and female partners	10 (23%)

TABLE 3. Sexual Risk Behaviors in the Last Six Months of Partners of MtF Transgendered Persons*

	Sex with Trans- gendered Partners: n (%)	Sex with Male Partners: n (%)	Sex with Female Partners: n (%)
Any type of sex	43 (100%)	16 (37%)	27 (63%)
Two or more partners*	25 (58%)	14 (88%)	18 (67%)
Insertive anal sex*	33 (77%)	11 (69%)	23 (85%)
Unprotected insertive anal sex**	19 (58%)	7 (64%)	19 (83%)
Receptive anal sex*	7 (16%)	3 (19%)	N/A
Unprotected receptive anal sex**	4 (57%)	2 (67%)	N/A
Insertive vaginal sex*	10 (23%)	N/A	23 (85%)
Unprotected insertive vaginal sex**	7 (70%)	N/A	19 (83%)

*Denominators for percentages listed represent the total number of participants reporting any type of sex.
**Denominators for percentages listed represent the total number of participants reporting the particular type of sex.

tected sex with both a transgendered partner and a female partner in the last six months.

Drug Use

Non-injection and injection drug use in the last three months were prevalent among the sample. The most common drugs reported are listed in Table 4. The top three drugs reported were alcohol (72%), marijuana (67%), and crack or cocaine (49%). Thirty percent (n = 13) had ever injected drugs, 77% (n = 10) of those who had ever injected had done so in the prior three months, and 40% (n = 4) of those who reported injecting drugs in the prior three months had shared needles.

HIV Awareness and Perceptions of Risk

Male participants indicated concern about the substantial high-risk behavior that they reported and seemed to perceive themselves to be at risk for HIV. When asked how concerned they were about HIV, 70% (n = 30) reported being somewhat or very concerned (Table 5). Twenty-one percent (n = 9) reported being only a little concerned or not at all concerned, and the remaining 9% (n = 4) did not know if they were concerned.

When asked why they were or were not concerned, HIV-negative respondents cited several reasons. The most common reasons for being concerned were that they perceived themselves to be at risk for acquiring HIV and they did not want to get sick or die. Further, nearly three-quarters of the sample (72%, n = 31) reported having received an HIV test at some point prior to taking the survey, which supports the notion that the men perceived themselves to be at risk. The main reason given for low levels of concern was that they practice safe sex.

Seven of the eight HIV-positive people said they were somewhat or very concerned. The primary reason for concern they mentioned was that they were concerned about the spread of HIV and did not want others to get it.

HIV-Positive Respondents

The eight HIV-positive respondents were asked the open-ended question, "What are the circumstances that led to you becoming HIV-positive? Tell me about how you think you got HIV." The purpose of this question was to explore transmission patterns, in addition to risk factors that could lead to possible transmission. Four respondents said that they contracted HIV through unprotected sex, three believed they got HIV from either unprotected sex or needle sharing, and one said he got HIV from a blood transfusion. One person mentioned his sexual

TABLE 4. Drug Use and Injection History of Male Partners of MtF Transgendered Persons

Drug Use and Injection	n (%)
Type of Drug Used in the Last Three Months	
Alcohol	31 (72%)
Marijuana	29 (67%)
Crack or cocaine	21 (49%)
Speed	11 (26%)
Poppers	6 (14%)
Injection History	
Ever injected drugs	13 (30%)
Injected in last three months	10 (77%)*
Shared needles in last three months	4 (40%)**

*Percent of those who ever injected
**Percent of those who injected in the last three months

TABLE 5. Level of Concern About HIV Among Male Partners of MtF Transgendered Persons

Response	All Participants		HIV-Positive Participants	
	n	%	n	%
Very concerned	21	49	4	50
Somewhat concerned	9	21	3	38
A little concerned	2	5	0	0
Not at all concerned	7	16	1	13
Do not know	4	9	0	0
Total	43	100	8	100

relationships with MtF persons as a possible way that he became infected, and another attributed the source of his infection to a male partner. A third person identified selling sex for money and drugs as a contributing factor.

Results from Focus Groups with MtF Transgendered Persons

Characteristics of Men Who Have Sex with Transgendered Persons

According to the focus group participants, there is no single "defining characteristic" of the male partners of MtF. As one participant said, "As far as what type, there is no type. They're all different sizes, shapes, and colors." Another participant spoke about her boyfriends: "Some were gigolos, which made me feel comfortable. . . . All the hustle was on my man." In contrast, another participant described her partner as a "typical" man. She explained, "I have a husband. I've been married two-and-a-half years. He's just a typical, ordinary man. He has a job, a house, money, he pays my rent."

Participants stated that their sex work clients are often married to biological women and of fairly high economic status. One participant commented, "A lot [of the sex work clients] have responsibilities at home—a wife, children. The men who go to transgenders for sex want their sex fantasy to happen. But they keep their family because in society family means you have security, stability. But they go around transgenders and will pay however much."

When focus group participants were asked about the sexual orientation of their boyfriends or husbands, many transgendered individuals described their long-term partners as heterosexual. One participant said, "I've been with a guy five years. Straight as can be. He definitely thinks of himself as straight." Another described how her partner's sexual orientation supports her gender identity: "[My boyfriend is] so very confident about his masculinity, and I would like to think of him as very straight . . . He makes me feel very womanly, so much of a woman."

Other participants, while agreeing that their male partners are not gay, viewed them as bisexual rather than heterosexual. For example, one participant responded, "They're not gay. They're more in the bisexual category because they're not attracted to men in pants. But they want the best of both worlds." Another explained why the men do not consider themselves gay, saying, "Almost all of them are bisexual but they don't categorize themselves as gay, because they would never like a guy who looks like a man."

Sexual Behavior

Many participants claimed that their male partners engage in anal receptive sex, despite the low reports of this type of sex among the male interview participants. As one transgendered participant stated, "The men who call themselves straight and say they'll never do that [bottom], they're lying. You never know what they'll do at some time, with some people." Another participant commented, "When they're going to have sex, in the heat of the moment, the excitement of the moment, they'll go for anything." According to focus groups participants, their male partners engage in anal receptive sex because they want sex that is different from the sex they have at home with their wives. "The sex with us they want to be totally different from at home. How can we make it different? By going up in it. Penetration." Some participants highlighted the relationship between sexual identity and having certain kinds of sex with transgendered persons. "Most [of our male partners] are bottoms—that's the weirdest thing because they're really masculine and not gay. They won't let men do it to them."

Other focus group participants had difficulty generalizing about whether their partners are more often "tops" (i.e., insertive partners) or "bottoms" (i.e., receptive partners). One participant commented, "A lot of them are tops, but sometimes they ask me if I'm functional. If they find out that I don't have a penis, they don't like me. Most are bottoms, but a lot are tops." Another felt that men engage in both behaviors. "Most are bottoms, most are tops. Any way they can get it."

Participants discussed the risk behavior that occurs with their male partners. One participant noted: "There's a lot of unprotected sex, but it's a whole realm of things." A number of participants contended that many men pay more to have unprotected sex. According to one transgendered individual, "They're the ones who encourage you not to use condoms. They give you more money not to." Another participant affirmed, "They will pay extra not to use a rubber–they'll be almost begging not to use it." Another agreed, "Most people I dated for sex for money, I don't get penetrated . . . but I can give it [penetration] to them if they want to pay more . . ."

Finally, focus group members made reference to the complex sexual networks of MtF persons and their male partners. In describing their male partners, some participants said that many transgendered individuals were having sex with the same men. One participant observed, "I've been in San Francisco 20 years. Most of the men bounce from one TG [transgendered person] to another."

Drug Use

Although focus group participants were not asked explicitly about drug use, transgendered individuals in both groups discussed the role that drug use plays in increasing the risk of HIV transmission. Some participants believed that their male partners use drugs to help them keep their sexual activity with transgendered individuals in the realm of fantasy. They reported that drugs help the men avoid the reality of their behavior and the reality of the health risks involved. "Even if they only hit the pipe once, for those 20 minutes it's their fantasy, their secret. They aren't concerned about that fantasy afterwards." Another participant held a similar opinion, saying: "They give into their impulse according to their sexual fantasy. Before they can think of protection, they want their fantasy ful-

filled. And most are involved in drugs. They use drugs to approach and accept themselves, that they have fantasies like that."

Focus group participants spoke specifically about the effects of smoking crack cocaine. They noted how it lowers their and their partners' inhibitions. "Most men when they smoke they want to get fucked. They say that's the only time they do it is when they smoke crack." Participants also indicated that crack use among their male partners affected their partners' disclosure of HIV status. One participant stated, "No, they never tell you. The drug takes over and it's on. Especially if it's crack."

DISCUSSION

Limitations

This needs assessment has a number of limitations that should be considered when reviewing and interpreting the results. First, the relatively small sample size and nonrandom sampling techniques prevent the generalization of findings to the larger population. Second, it is possible that economic necessity may have led some male survey respondents to claim they have sex with MtF persons in order to receive the cash incentive, although every effort was made to screen potential participants well and no one was denied the cash incentive if it was determined during the survey that they did not have MtF sexual partners. In addition, the survey data are generally consistent with the limited research on the male partners of MtF, further supporting the validity of the survey data. Finally, the survey explored sex-related risks in much greater depth than drug-related risks, and thus cannot be considered an exhaustive assessment of risk.

Discussion

Looking at the findings from the interviews and focus groups together, five main themes with direct implications for HIV prevention are apparent. First, our findings suggest that male partners of MtF persons do not have a distinct profile–they are of all ages, races, sexual orientations, and socioeconomic backgrounds.

Second, high-risk sex occurs between MtF persons and their sexual partners, despite high levels of concern reported among both male and MtF participants. The data suggest that both MtF persons and their male partners could be at high risk for acquiring HIV, depending on the serostatus of their partners, since both report unprotected receptive anal sex. Further, a study completed in Brazil found that among MtF sex workers, engaging in insertive anal sex with men was a significant predictor of HIV infection.[13] This finding raises a concern regarding the risk among heterosexually identified men, a group that is not considered to be at high risk in San Francisco. Nevertheless, two of the HIV-positive interview participants identified as heterosexual, which suggests that HIV prevention resources for this subgroup of heterosexual men may be warranted.

Third, drug use appears to play a role in unsafe sex, especially in situations in which sex is exchanged for drugs or money. Crack use, in particular, was cited in the focus groups as a drug that can lower inhibitions and contribute to engaging in high-risk behaviors.

Fourth, the male partners of MtF may represent a possible bridge for HIV transmission among different populations, given that they reported unprotected sex with male and female partners, as well as transgendered partners. In this study, two men reported unprotected sex with both an MtF and a female partner in the last six months.

Finally, receptive anal sex, one of the highest risk behaviors for HIV transmission, was reported infrequently by male participants. In contrast, MtF participants reported that men frequently engage in this type of sex with them. A likely explanation for this discrepancy is that the men under-reported this behavior, due to internalized homophobia and the particular stigma associated with this type of sex.

Until recently, HIV prevention resources have been almost exclusively directed at HIV-negative individuals, and program messages have centered on how to protect oneself from acquiring HIV. In the past few years, "prevention for positives" programs have received increased funding, and for the first time in San Francisco, funding for services that support HIV-positive individuals in preventing the spread of HIV was prioritized.[1] This needs assessment is an example of research that focuses on the sexual partners of a high-prevalence, high-incidence population so that appropriate interventions can be developed, not only to prevent HIV-negative men who have sex with MtF from becoming infected, but also to support male partners who are HIV-positive or of unknown serostatus in preventing transmission to others.

Targeting prevention efforts at the male partners of MtF individuals will be challenging. They are a hidden population because of the stigma associated with sex with MtF, and thus they do not have a community in which prevention messages can be disseminated, such as gay men have. Further, many identify as heterosexual and thus would be missed by existing prevention efforts in San Francisco, where heterosexual transmission is low and few resources address the non-injection drug using heterosexual population.

However, MtF transgendered individuals are in a unique position to reach this population (their male partners), and we recommend that they be included in any efforts to plan and implement HIV prevention activities with their male partners. It is also critical for community-based prevention to address some of the underlying social and economic issues that affect MtF and their male partners. Without attention to the economic insecurity, mental health, and substance use issues among both MtF individuals and their male partners, prevention efforts will have limited if any effectiveness.

Further research assessing the size of the population of men who have sex with transgendered persons, as well as the extent of HIV risk behaviors among MtF, their male partners, and their sexual networks beyond the small sample in this study, may be helpful for determining the appropriate level of HIV prevention resources.

REFERENCES

1. 2001 San Francisco HIV Prevention Plan. http://www.dph.sf.ca.us/HIVPrevPlan/page2.htm.

2. Clements-Nolle K., Marx R., Guzman R., Katz M. (2001) HIV prevalence, risk behaviors, health care use, and mental health status of transgender persons: Implications for public health intervention. Am J Public Health 91(6):915-921.

3. Kellogg T.A., Clements-Nolle K., Dilley J., Katz M.H., McFarland W. (2001) Incidence of human immunodeficiency virus among male-to-female transgendered persons in San Francisco. J Acquir Immune Defic Syndr 28(4): 380-384.

4. Hooley J. (1996) The Transgender Project. Sydney: Central Sydney Area Health Service.

5. Bockting W.O., Robinson B.E., Rosser B.R.S. (1998) Transgender HIV prevention: A qualitative needs assessment. AIDS Care 10(4):505-526.

6. McGowan C.K. (2000) Transgender needs assessment. New York: The City of New York Department of Health.

7. Mason T.H. (1995) Gender identity support services for transgenders: Beacon Hill Multicultural Psychological Association, prepared for the Massachusetts Department of Public Health HIV/AIDS Bureau.

8. Boles J., Elifson K. (1994) The social organization of transvestite prostitution and AIDS. Soc Sci Med 39(1): 85-93.

9. Weinberg M.S. (1999) Gendered sex work in the San Francisco Tenderloin. Arch Sex Behav 28(6):503-521.

10. Perkins R., Griffin A., Jakobsen J. (1994) Lifestyles and HIV/AIDS risk: National transgender HIV/AIDS needs assessment project. New South Wales, Australia: School of Sociology, University of New South Wales.

11. Because an early screening question asking about sex with transgendered persons seemed too intrusive, questions about sex with transgendered persons did not appear until about halfway through the questionnaire. This explains the high percentage of ineligible men who nevertheless were interviewed.

12. Inciardi J.A., Surratt H.L., Telles P.R., Pok B.H. (1999) Sex, drugs, and the culture of transvestimo in Rio de Jainero. *IJT* 3(1+2), http://www.symposion.com/ijt/hiv_risk/inciardi.htm.

13. SPSS Inc., Chicago, IL, http://www.spss.com/.

A Needs Assessment of Transgendered People of Color Living in Washington, DC

Jessica M. Xavier, MPH
Marilyn Bobbin, MBA, MS, RD
Ben Singer, PhD candidate
Earline Budd

SUMMARY. A needs assessment (N = 248) conducted in Washington, DC, revealed that transgendered people of color are at high risk for HIV/AIDS, substance abuse, suicide and violence/crime victimization. Overall HIV prevalence was 25%, with 32% in natal males (MTFs, i.e., male-to-females). Four predictors for HIV positive status were identified through logistic regression–male sex at birth, a history of substance abuse, sexual assault, and unemployment. Substance abuse was found in nearly half the sample (48%) but only half of those (51%) had sought treatment for it. Thirty-eight percent reported experiencing suicidal ideation, with 63% of those attributing it to their gender issues. Of those with suicidal ideation, nearly half (49%, or 16% of the entire sample), went on to make attempt(s) to kill themselves. Forty-three percent had been victims of violence or crime, including 13% who had been sexually assaulted.

Knowledge of the *Standards of Care* of the Harry Benjamin International Gender Dysphoria Association was quite low (9%) and associated with white race, any higher education beyond high school, and access to sex reassignment surgery (SRS). Access to SRS, defined as obtaining vaginoplasties for natal males and chest surgeries for natal females, was just 4%. White race (versus all other races, p < .001) and female at birth (versus male, p < .01) were significantly associated with access to SRS.

Use of hormones at some point during their lives was reported by 51% of participants. Thirty-five percent were currently taking hormones, with 72% acquiring their hormones from friends or on the street. Among natal males, 25% had injected silicone.

Jessica M. Xavier, MPH, is affiliated with Transresearch.org. Marilyn Bobbin, MBA, MS, RD, resides in College Park, MD. Ben Singer, PhD candidate, is affiliated with GenderWorks Consulting Group. Earline Budd is affiliated with Transgender Health Empowerment, Inc.

Address correspondence to: Jessica M. Xavier, P.O. Box 65, Kensington, MD 20895 (E-mail: jessicax@ earthlink.net).

The authors would like to express their gratitude to Ron Simmons, PhD, and R. Cameron Wolf, PhD, MS, for their invaluable contributions to the administration and prior analysis of the Washington, DC Transgender Needs Assessment Survey (WTNAS), and Emilia Lombardi, PhD, for her review of this paper.

Funding for the WTNAS was provided by the HIV and AIDS Administration of the District of Columbia Government, through Us Helping Us–People Into Living, Inc.

In memory of Tina Teasley, Pat Hamilton, Jean Robinson-Bay, Sparkle Maharis, Jeffrey Pendleton, Tyra Hunter, Stephanie Thomas, Ukea Davis, and many others no longer with us, who dared to express a different gender in the District of Columbia.

[Haworth co-indexing entry note]: "A Needs Assessment of Transgendered People of Color Living in Washington, DC." Xavier, Jessica M. et al. Co-published simultaneously in *International Journal of Transgenderism* (The Haworth Medical Press, an imprint of The Haworth Press, Inc.) Vol. 8, No. 2/3, 2005, pp. 31-47; and: *Transgender Health and HIV Prevention: Needs Assessment Studies from Transgender Communities Across the United States* (ed: Walter Bockting, and Eric Avery) The Haworth Medical Press, an imprint of The Haworth Press, Inc., 2005, pp. 31-47. Single or multiple copies of this article are available for a fee from The Haworth Document Delivery Service [1-800-HAWORTH, 9:00 a.m. - 5:00 p.m. (EST). E-mail address: docdelivery@haworthpress.com].

Nineteen percent did not have their own living space, and employment, housing and job training were the most commonly-reported immediate needs of the sample. The results of this needs assessment provide evidence of an urgent need for increased medical and social services specific to transgendered people of color living in the District of Columbia. *[Article copies available for a fee from The Haworth Document Delivery Service: 1-800-HAWORTH. E-mail address: <docdelivery@haworthpress.com> Website: <http://www.HaworthPress.com> © 2005 by The Haworth Press, Inc. All rights reserved.]*

KEYWORDS. Transgender people of color, African American, Hispanic, HIV/AIDS, health and social services

INTRODUCTION

Washington, DC, has one of the highest per capita AIDS prevalence rates in the United States. As of June 2001, that prevalence rate was 166 cases per 100,000 population–more than eleven times the national average.[1] Over 6,832 people are living with AIDS in the District of Columbia, and 17,000 others are infected with HIV. Nearly one out of every twenty adult residents of the Nation's Capital is HIV positive.

Despite well quantified data on HIV infection in other at-risk subgroups in the District,[2] little has been known about rates of infection among its transgendered population. Transgendered people are those who cannot or choose not to conform to societal gender norms based upon their physical or birth sex. Transgendered people living in the District are likely its most heavily stigmatized, socially marginalized and with regard to HIV/AIDS, perpetually underserved, at-risk population. The DC Department of Health has traditionally included them in the same educational and prevention categories and modalities as men who have sex with men (MSM), which may explain the lack of culturally appropriate HIV prevention services available to them. Studies in other cities[3,4,5] have found that existing MSM prevention methods are not inclusive of transgendered individuals and are ineffective for them. In 1999, the American Public Health Association recommended that the health care needs of MTF and FTM transgendered people be considered as separate and distinct from those of gay men and lesbians.[6] The *Healthy People 2010 Companion Document for Lesbian, Gay, Bisexual, and Transgender Health* stresses that understanding the psychosocial complexities of a given

at-risk population is a key factor in developing culturally-appropriate education and prevention materials, and further suggests that cultural competency for health care agencies and providers working with lesbian, gay, bisexual and transgendered people is essential for successful interventions.[7]

Transgendered people have been difficult to study for a variety of reasons. Social stigma places many if not most transgendered people at society's margins, and many will not disclose their transgendered status for fear of violence and discrimination.[3] Hence, prevalence data are scarce. In San Francisco, a city well known for having a large sexual minority population, estimates of the number of transgendered residents ranged from 6,000-7,000 in 1994[8] to 22,000 in 2001, or 0.7% to 2.2% of its total population.[9] Unlike San Francisco's transgendered community, which has a large, visible, sustained system of supportive organizations and public health service providers, Washington, DC's smaller transgendered population remains largely isolated.

In addition to their marginalization, transgendered people use a variety of self-descriptive identity terms that defy precise categorization in most data collection instruments. As in diverse populations of MSM, transgendered persons vary widely along cultural, racial, ethnic and class lines. Broadly speaking, there are two principal gender vectors: natal males with female identification or expression (male-to-females, or MTFs) and natal females with male identification or expression (female-to-males, or FTMs). In addition, there are many visibly gender variant gay, lesbian and bisexual people who do not self-identify as transgender. Self-identification has hampered other efforts at studying gender variant persons who only identify as gay, lesbian, or bisexual, or do not use the term transgender to self-identify. As a result, significant numbers of transgender or transgender-appearing people may be unintentionally omitted from many research efforts.

Transgendered people living in the District of Columbia are a difficult to define, heavily stigmatized, and socially marginalized population. They are divided along racial, class, gender vector and full-time living status, while living under the aggregate oppressions of gender, race and class. The combined impact of all these factors has resulted in the lack of organized advocacy for health care and social services and no definitive research to define the needs of this population. Addition of mortality and morbidity factors brought on by HIV/AIDS and other sexually transmitted diseases (STDs), substance abuse, malnutrition, violence, homelessness, chronic mental health issues such as depression and gender dysphoria all combine to paint a picture of perhaps the single-most desperate population in the District.

Public health interventions demand hard data, which has been difficult to obtain in this population for the aforementioned reasons. Moreover, with the exception of a few courageous individuals during the late 1980s and early 1990s, there has been very little in the way of organized efforts by openly transgendered persons to advocate for research, education and prevention, cultural sensitivity training, and outreach efforts within the District of Columbia. The purpose of the research presented in this article has been to close the information gap around transgendered residents of the District by documenting the health disparities that put them at need for life-saving health and social services.

METHODS

In order to document the needs and concerns of transgendered residents of the District, a community-based research initiative began in 1998, evolving into the Washington, DC Transgender Needs Assessment Survey (WTNAS)–the largest quantitative study of an urban transgender population conducted to date on the eastern coast of the United States. The HIV and AIDS Administration of the District of Columbia Department of Health agreed to fund the survey after a short but intensive period of advocacy for its implementation. The primary goal of the WTNAS was to provide the District Government, community-based social service organizations, and AIDS Service Organizations with the first in-depth analysis of the health and housing concerns of the District's transgendered residents. Its data and recommendations will assist these agencies in specifically targeting and allocating intervention services for transgendered people in need. While the earliest HIV risk studies done in the U.S.[10,11] focused on MTF transgender sex workers, it was deemed more important to collect survey data that reflected the needs, issues and concerns of the majority transgendered population of Washington. Moreover, earlier research suggests that interrelated factors such as the sociodemographics, housing, and general and transgender-related health care issues of transgendered people have a direct impact on their HIV status, their safer sex practices and their access to both HIV education and prevention efforts and HIV-related care.

Rather than limit participation to only self-identified transgendered people, eligibility for the survey was open to anyone who was a resident of the District of Columbia, visibly gender variant and willing to give signed informed consent. Gender variant people were defined as those who live or want to live full-time in a gender opposite their birth or physical sex; those who have or want to physically modify their bodies to match their internal gender identity; and those who wear the clothing of the opposite sex in order to fully express an inner, cross-gender identity.

Annual income was asked without regard to household income. In order to capture the sizeable numbers of Latino/a transgendered people, the survey questionnaire was translated into Spanish for their use. The majority of the youth who participated were interviewed at the Sexual Minority Youth Assistance League (SMYAL), with the full cooperation of that agency. In addition to a sequential number, each questionnaire was assigned an acrostic–a unique identifier for each participant, using parts of the first and last names and date of birth–in order to prevent duplication.

Many cases of national and international anti-transgender violence have been reported through *Remembering Our Dead*,[12] a web-based project of Gender Education & Advocacy, Inc. The survey's questions regarding violence and crime victimization, as well as perceived motives, were taken from the standard form of the National Coalition of Anti-Violence Programs (NCAVP) used by its participating organizations throughout the U.S. to report bias-related crimes committed against gay, lesbian, bisexual, and transgender persons, as well as persons living with AIDS.[13]

Access to care is defined here as successfully obtaining a medical or non-medical procedure or service, either through licensed providers or illicit means. We measured access on a lifetime basis for regular health care, transgender-related care and HIV-related care, using Likert scales rating quality of service and provider sensitivity to the transgendered participant. Only those participants who had actually accessed a service were asked to rate it. Regular health care services were defined as exclusive of the other two categories, and included routine medical screening (for high blood pressure, high cholesterol, cancer, etc.), dental care, vision care and urgent medical care. Some transgender-related services or types of care were accessed by the participants through licensed medical providers and/or illicit means. Since many transgendered persons seek to alter their bodies in varying degrees to achieve some measure of congruency with their internal gender identity, their anatomy is often in flux. Consequently, an anatomy inventory was included in the survey to assess the degree to which the participants had accessed various surgical, cosmetic and hormonal procedures. Injection Silicone Use (ISU) is defined here as receiving or self-administering injections of silicone or other heavy oils in the cheeks, breasts, hips and buttocks.

Due to the scope of the survey, we limited assessment of behavioral health to only substance abuse and suicide issues. Apart from self-reporting an alcohol or drug problem, we did not ask the participants about their specific drug use, nor did we specify the purpose of injection use when asking about sharing needles. However, in addition to substance abuse and HIV, Hepatitis B and C transmission risks of Injection Drug Use (IDU), transgender people face systemic health risks for Injection Silicone Use (ISU) and viral transmission risks in injection hormone use when needles are shared.

While some earlier research of urban U.S. transgender populations[4,10,11] also discussed HIV/STD risks in countries other than the U.S.,[14,15,16] we felt it important to restrict our discussion only to other U.S. transgender populations. There are profound differences between American transgendered populations and those in other countries, with regard to culture, language, degree of social acceptance, and the presence (or lack) of a national health care system.

HIV status was self-reported by the participants. Participants also reported their specific sexual risk behaviors associated with the transmission of HIV and other sexually-transmitted diseases. The participants indicated whether they had engaged in a specific risk behavior at least once in the last month, at least once in the last year, at least once during their lives, or never. In order to make the risk behaviors applicable to both gender vectors (MTF/FTM), and due to the extreme sensitivity of many transgendered people with regard to their genitalia, explicit anatomical terms were avoided, and general terms ("genital," "oral," "anal," "manual," etc.) were used wherever possible in the behavioral risk descriptions.

Due to the variety of self-identification terms used by the participants of the survey, we analyzed differences between natal males and natal females. More specifically, we examined the associations between various lifetime sociodemographic variables and HIV positive status, and specific risk factors and HIV positive status using a Chi-Square, two-sided, at alpha = .05. We then developed a logistic regression model to identify the predictors of HIV positive status, with all variables tested shown in Table 7. Only p-values significant at .05 are reported.

We recruited participants using convenience sampling, snowball technique with a financial incentive of $10 to participate. Key members of transgender subpopulations were identified and recruited as survey administrators. Nearly all of the participants were invited to participate by survey administrators through their memberships in transgender support groups, their social networks, or their paid or volunteer outreach work conducted by several different AIDS Service Organizations located in the District.

Of the twelve trained survey administrators, ten identified themselves as transgender, and seven were of color. All signed confidentiality statements, in which they promised to safeguard the privacy of all WTNAS participants. Ultimately, nine survey administrators were involved in successful data collection. The survey administrators as well as the participants were paid for their efforts in this survey. Data collection for the WTNAS began on September 18, 1999, and was completed on January 31, 2000, with a total of 252 completed, unduplicated questionnaires collected during that period. The initial results were presented in the survey's final report.[17] For this analysis, the data were analyzed using SPSS 10 for Windows. Due to our analytical focus on natal sex status, four intersexed persons in the original sample were excluded, leaving a total of 248 participants.

RESULTS

Sociodemographics

Table 1 presents the sociodemographic characteristics of the sample, broken down by natal sex status. Among the 248 participants of this

TABLE 1. Demographics of the WTNAS Sample, Washington, DC, 1999-2000 (n = 248)

	ALL PARTICIPANTS (n = 248)	NATAL MALES (n = 188)	NATAL FEMALES (n = 60)
AGE RANGE			
13 to 19	54 (22%)	29 (15%)	25 (42%)
20 to 24	43 (17%)	39 (21%)	4 (7%)
25 to 29	51 (21%)	45 (24%)	6 (10%)
30 to 39	58 (23%)	47 (25%)	11 (18%)
40 to 49	34 (14%)	25 (13%)	9 (15%)
50 to 59	7 (3%)	3 (2%)	4 (7%)
60 to 61	1	0	1 (1%)
Median Age	27	27	26
GENDER IDENTITY			
Man	30 (12%)	23 (12%)	7 (12%)
Woman	35 (14%)	12 (6%)	23 (38%)
Transgender	174 (70%)	147 (78%)	27 (45%)
Other	9 (4%)	6 (3%)	3 (5%)
RACE			
African American	174 (70%)	129 (68%)	45 (75%)
Hispanic-Latino/a	53 (21%)	52 (28%)	1 (1%)
White	10 (4%)	3 (2%)	7 (12%)
Other	11 (5%)	4 (2%)	7 (12%)
SEXUAL ORIENTATION			
Heterosexual	8 (3%)	7 (4%)	1 (1%)
Gay	164 (66%)	148 (79%)	16 (27%)
Lesbian	29 (12%)	2 (1%)	27 (45%)
Bisexual	32 (13%)	21 (11%)	11 (18%)
Other	15 (6%)	10 (5%)	5 (8%)
EDUCATION (not including youth aged 13-19)			
Less than High School	59 (30%)	56 (35%)	3 (9%)
HS/GED/Tech School	65 (34%)	53 (33%)	12 (34%)
Any Higher Education	70 (36%)	50 (31%)	20 (57%)
EMPLOYMENT (not including youth aged 13-19)			
Employed	126 (65%)	99 (63%)	27 (77%)
Unemployed	67 (35%)	59 (37%)	8 (23%)
ANNUAL INCOME (not including youth aged 13-19)			
< $15,000	123 (64%)	114 (73%)	9 (26%)
$15,000 +	68 (36%)	42 (27%)	26 (74%)

sample, 188 (76%) were natal males and 60 (24%) were natal females (p < .001). They ranged in age from 13 to 61, with a mean age of 29 years and standard deviation of 9.79. The predominant gender identity of all participants was transgender (69%), with 65% reporting their sexual orientation as gay. The majority (69%) reported their relationship status as single. Over 94% of the participants in the sample were of color (either African-American, Latino-American, Native-American, or biracial/multiracial) with 70% African-American. English was the most commonly-spoken language (76%), followed by Spanish (13%). Twenty-three of the participants (9%) were bilingual, with the majority of those (n = 20) bilingual in English and Spanish. Two hundred nine participants (84%) were U.S. citizens, and 19% had immigrated to the U.S., mostly from Latin American countries, with the majority having immigrated from El Salvador (n = 17) and Mexico (n = 7).

After removing youth (participants aged 13-19) from the analysis, 30% of the adult participants did not finish High School or possess a GED, 35% were unemployed and 64% reported their annual income as less than $15,000. The most common barriers to employment among unemployed adults were discrimination based upon transgendered status or gender variant appearance (34%) and disability (33%). In the entire sample, 15% reported job loss from discrimination, with natal males more likely to have lost their employment than natal females (p < .05).

Violence and Crime Victimization

One hundred seven participants (43%) had been victims of violence or crime. Thirteen percent had been victims of sexual assault or rape, including 12% of the natal males and 18% of the natal females. The victims perceived the most common motives for the violence to be homophobia (43%) and transphobia (35%).

Access to Regular Health Care Services

Although those who accessed regular medical services indicated high levels of satisfaction in both areas, overall access was low (Table 2). Just 9% reported specific difficulties accessing regular health care services, with the most commonly-reported barriers to access being no health insurance (68%), inability to pay (48%), caregiver insensitivity or hostility to transgendered people (33%), and fear of disclosure of transgender status (33%).

Almost half of the participants (47%) did not have health insurance, and 40% reported not having a doctor whom they saw for regular health care. Natal males were more likely to lack health insurance (58% vs. 15% of natal females, p < .001). Natal males were more likely to access DC Emergency Medical Services (ambulance) than natal females (p < .01) while natal females were more likely to obtain vision

TABLE 2. Lifetime Level of Access to Regular Health Care Services

REGULAR HEALTH CARE SERVICE	OVERALL ACCESS	ACCESS BY NATAL MALES	ACCESS BY NATAL FEMALES	P VALUES
Annual Physical Exam with Blood Work	135 (54%)	100 (53%)	35 (58%)	
Routine Prescriptions	107 (43%)	75 (40%)	32 (53%)	
Dental Care	98 (40%)	76 (40%)	22 (37%)	
Routine Medical Screening	88 (36%)	68 (36%)	20 (33%)	
Emergency Room Visits	74 (30%)	59 (31%)	15 (25%)	
DC Emergency Medical Services	67 (27%)	59 (31%)	8 (13%)	p < .01
Vision Care	57 (23%)	37 (20%)	20 (33%)	p < .05
Routine Hospitalization	53 (21%)	40 (21%)	13 (22%)	
Specialist Care	32 (13%)	21 (11%)	11 (8%)	
Gynecological Care	25 (10%)	3 (2%)	22 (37%)	p < .001

care ($p < .05$) and gynecological care ($p < .001$). However, only a little more than a third of the natal females had had a gynecological exam in their lifetimes.

Access to Transgender-Related Health Care

Despite high reported levels of satisfaction with access to transgender-related care by the participants on a lifetime basis, overall access was low, with the exception of access to psychotherapy and hormone prescriptions (Table 3). However, only 11% reported specific difficulties accessing transgender-related health care services. The barriers most frequently reported were inability to pay (50%), not knowing where to obtain services (35%), health insurers' denial of coverage (31%), and provider insensitivity or hostility (31%). The most common sources of information about transgender health care for the participants were word of mouth (73%), gay newspapers (39%), transgender support groups (38%), and transgender newsletters or magazines (31%).

Using a limited definition of sex reassignment surgery (SRS) as obtaining vaginoplasties for natal males and chest surgeries for natal females, we found that only nine participants (4%) had undergone SRS. White race was significantly associated with access to SRS (50% of whites vs. 2% of all other races, $p < .001$) and natal females were more likely to undergo SRS (10% vs. 2% of the natal males, $p < .01$). None of the natal females had undergone breast reduction, metaoidioplasty, phalloplasty or clitoral release procedures.

After psychotherapy, hormone usage was the most commonly reported type of transgender-related health care accessed by the participants. Compared to natal females, natal males were more likely to obtain hormone prescriptions (27% vs. 12%, $p < .05$). Among natal males, 25% had received silicone injections, which are viewed as a fast, cheap alternative to hormonal therapy that preserves sexual virility.

Fifty-one percent had taken hormones at least once, but only 33% reported that a doctor monitored their blood levels while receiving them. At the time of the survey, 35% of participants were taking hormones, and nearly all of them planned on taking them for the rest of their lives. However, 70% of those currently taking hormones had acquired them from friends or on the street, with natal males more likely than na-

TABLE 3. Level of Access to Transgender-Related Health Care Services

HEALTH CARE SERVICE/PROCEDURE	OVERALL ACCESS	ACCESS BY NATAL MALES	ACCESS BY NATAL FEMALES	P VALUES
Transgender-Related Psychotherapy	78 (32%)	57 (30%)	21 (35%)	
Hormone Prescriptions	58 (23%)	51 (27%)	7 (12%)	p < .05
Electrolysis	18 (7%)	17 (9%)	1 (2%)	
Hair Transplantation	2 (1%)	1 (< 1%)	1 (2%)	
Silicone Injections–Breasts/Face/Hips/Buttocks		47 (25%)		
Facial Cosmetic Surgery		10 (5.3%)		
Saline Breast Implants		5 (3%)		
Speech Therapy		5 (3%)		
Vaginoplasty		3 (2%)		
Liposuction		3 (2%)		
Silicone Breast Implants		2 (1%)		
Tracheal Procedure		2 (1%)		
Labiaplasty		2 (1%)		
Vocal Cord Surgery		1 (< 1%)		
Orchiectomy		1 (< 1%)		
FTM Chest Surgery			6 (10%)	
Hysterectomy			3 (5%)	
Oophorectomy			6 (10%)	
Vaginectomy			1 (2%)	

tal females (74% vs. 25%, p <.01) to do so. Natal females were more likely than natal males to get their hormone levels monitored (88% vs. 29%, p = .001). Of those who had never taken hormones, 18% were planning to take them in the future.

Anatomical Inventory

Results of the natal and altered anatomy inventories are listed in Table 4. In many cases, participants did not report gonadal genitalia, which accounts for smaller numbers of testicles, uteruses and ovaries.

The most commonly-known means for governing access to hormonal therapy and surgical sex reassignment is the *Standards of Care* (*SOC*) published by the Harry Benjamin International Gender Dysphoria Association (HBIGDA).[18] Only 9% of all participants were familiar with the *SOC*, with natal females more likely than natal males to know about them (p < .001). White race, any education beyond high school and access to sex reassignment surgery also were associated with knowledge of the *SOC* (all p < .001). For the participants who knew about the *SOC* (n = 22), only slightly more than half (54%) of their transgender health care providers had mentioned the *SOC* during their course of treatment. Thirty-five percent of the participants had to educate their medical or mental health providers about their needs as a transgendered person.

Housing Issues

Two hundred participants (81%) responded that they had their own living space, defined as at least a room of their own, and the majority of them lived with at least one other person. Natal females were more likely to have their own living space (95% vs. 76% of natal males, p <.01). Nineteen percent did not have their own living space, and the most common barriers to housing were economic situation, housing staff insensitivity or hostility to transgendered people, estrangement from birth family, and lack of employment. Nineteen percent had been evicted during their lifetimes, with the most common reasons cited for evictions being inability to pay the rent and substance abuse issues.

Substance Abuse and Suicidal Ideation/ Attempts

Nearly half the sample (110 participants, or 48%) reported a substance abuse problem with alcohol and/or non-specific drugs. Forty-seven percent reported having sex while drunk or high. Twenty-two percent admitted their drug use was a reason for having unsafe sex, and 9% had unsafe sex to obtain drugs. Substance abuse was also associated with sex work (p < .05). Only 36% of those with alcohol problems and 53% of those with drug problems sought treatment for them. We also found that substance abuse was associated with sex work (p < .05).

Thirty-eight percent reported experiencing suicidal ideation during their lifetimes, with 63% of those attributing it to their gender issues. Natal females were more likely to report suicidal ideation (52% vs. 33% in natal males, p < .05), but natal males were more likely to attribute their suicidal ideation to their gender issues (79% vs. 36%, p < .001). By age group, 41% of youth (13-19) reported suicidal ideation, followed by 18% of those 20-29, then 52% for those aged 30 and above (p < .001).

TABLE 4. Natal and Altered Anatomy Inventory

NATAL ANATOMY TYPE	NATAL MALES (n = 188)	NATAL FEMALES (n = 60)
Natal penis	182 (97%)	
Natal testicles	144 (77%)	
Natal vagina		59 (98%)
Natal clitoris		55 (92%)
Natal uterus		52 (87%)
Natal breasts		51 (85%)
Natal ovaries		48 (80%)
ALTERED ANATOMY TYPE		
Breasts through hormonal therapy	89 (47%)	
Breasts through silicone injections	25 (13%)	
Breasts with surgical implants	6 (3%)	
Surgically-constructed vagina	3 (2%)	
Surgically-constructed clitoris	3 (2%)	
Surgically-constructed labia	2 (1%)	
Hormonally-enlarged FTM genitalia		7 (12%)
Complete FTM chest surgery		6 (10%)

Controlling for other races, African-Americans were least likely to report suicidal ideation (p < .05). Of those with suicidal ideation, 49% (16% of the entire sample) made actual attempt(s) to kill themselves.

HIV Testing

Among all participants, 78% had been tested at least once for HIV. The majority (56%) of those who were not HIV positive reported getting tested either every six months or once a year; 19% of them had never been tested (14% of the overall sample). Natal males were more likely to get tested than natal females (78% vs. 22%, p < .05) and among the races, Latino/as were more likely than all other races to get tested (98% vs. 83%, p < .01). Testing was more common within the older age ranges, and 88% of those who admitted to at least one risky sexual behavior did get tested (p < .01). The most common reasons for participants not knowing their HIV status were feeling healthy, always having safer sex, or not wanting to know.

HIV Positive Participants and HIV/AIDS Services

Twenty-five percent of all participants reported being HIV positive, with another 22% who did not know their HIV status. Natal males were more likely than natal females to be HIV positive (32% vs. 3%, p < .001). Among those who reported being HIV positive, 72% had been diagnosed more than two years ago, and two-thirds believed they became infected with HIV through unprotected sex with non-transgendered males (68% vs. 32% for all other transmission factors combined, p < .001). Only four HIV positive participants (7%) encountered barriers to receiving HIV/AIDS services, with the most common barrier being provider insensitivity or hostility. The HIV positive participants generally reported high levels of satisfaction with the quality and sensitivity of HIV-related services they received.

HIV Risk Behaviors

The risk behaviors are listed in highest ranking order in Table 5. Overall, on a lifetime ba-

sis, 89% of the sample admitted to at least one unsafe behavior.

The most common reasons given by the participants who admitted to unsafe behaviors were they trusted their sex partner, their partner(s) appeared to be healthy, and they didn't know there was a risk associated with the behavior. Additionally, 4% of the participants had received a blood transfusion or other blood product at least once in their lifetimes. Although sharing of unclean needles for injection was low overall (4%), sharing uncleaned needles was associated with HIV positive status (p < .001); 13% of those who were HIV positive reported sharing uncleaned needles at least once.

Factors Associated with HIV-Positive Status

We tested a group of variables that would likely be associated with HIV positive status, with the bivariate results presented in Table 6. A subset of sociodemographic variables were entered into a logistic regression model, with the results presented in Table 7. Sexual orientation, education, suicide, and other risk factors were tested, yet were not significant.

Demand for Specific Services and Self-Assessment of Most Immediate Needs

To assess the demand for transgender-specific and transgender-sensitive services, all participants were asked to review a list of services and choose which they would be likely use if the services were available to them (Table 8). To assess their most pressing concerns, all participants were asked to identify the three most important, immediate needs which proved to be employment, housing and job training (Table 9).

In assessing the demand for transgender-specific or sensitive services, natal males were more likely than natal females to indicate their need to access hormone prescriptions, case management services, vocational training, substance abuse treatment, hotline or crisis intervention, transportation assistance (all p < .001), transgender-sensitive legal services (p < .01), and transgender health care information (p < .05), if they were available to them. Natal males were more likely than natal females to identify

TABLE 5. HIV Risk Behaviors

BEHAVIOR	PREVALENCE	ALL PARTICIPANTS	NATAL MALES	NATAL FEMALES	P VALUES
Unprotected Oral-Genital Contact	Cumulative (Lifetime)	191 (78%)	150 (82%)	41 (68%)	p < .05
	In the Last Month	89 (37%)	71 (38%)	18 (30%)	
	In the Last Year	51 (21%)	37 (20%)	14 (23%)	
	At Least Once	51 (21%)	42 (23%)	9 (15%)	
	Never	53 (22%)	34 (19%)	19 (32%)	
Unprotected Manual-Genital Contact	Cumulative (Lifetime)	188 (78%)	147 (81%)	41 (68%)	p < .05
	In the Last Month	104 (43%)	83 (46%)	21 (35%)	
	In the Last Year	42 (17%)	33 (18%)	9 (15%)	
	At Least Once	42 (17%)	31 (17%)	11 (18%)	
	Never	54 (22%)	35 (19%)	19 (32%)	
Unprotected Genital-Genital Contact	Cumulative (Lifetime)	166 (68%)	126 (69%)	40 (67%)	N.S.
	In the Last Month	48 (20%)	35 (19%)	13 (22%)	
	In the Last Year	46 (19%)	36 (21%)	8 (13%)	
	At Least Once	72 (30%)	53 (29%)	19 (32%)	
	Never	77 (32%)	57 (31%)	20 (33%)	
Sex While Inebriated	Cumulative (Lifetime)	115 (47%)	91 (49%)	24 (40%)	N.S.
	In the Last Month	40 (16%)	37 (20%)	3 (5%)	
	In the Last Year	36 (15%)	27 (15%)	9 (15%)	
	At Least Once	39 (16%)	27 (15%)	12 (20%)	
	Never	130 (53%)	94 (51%)	36 (60%)	
Unprotected Oral-Anal Contact	Cumulative (Lifetime)	108 (45%)	91 (50%)	17 (29%)	p < .01
	In the Last Month	45 (18%)	38 (21%)	7 (12%)	
	In the Last Year	34 (14%)	29 (16%)	5 (9%)	
	At Least Once	29 (12%)	24 (13%)	5 (9%)	
	Never	134 (55%)	92 (50%)	42 (71%)	
Unprotected Genital-Anal Contact	Cumulative (Lifetime)	105 (54%)	96 (72%)	9 (15%)	p < .001
	In the Last Month	27 (14%)	25 (19%)	2 (3%)	
	In the Last Year	35 (18%)	31 (23%)	4 (7%)	
	At Least Once	43 (22%)	40 (30%)	3 (5%)	
	Never	88 (46%)	38 (28%)	50 (85%)	
Unprotected Fisting	Cumulative (Lifetime)	47 (20%)	37 (21%)	10 (17%)	N.S.
	In the Last Month	20 (8%)	18 (10%)	2 (3%)	
	In the Last Year	16 (7%)	13 (7%)	3 (5%)	
	At Least Once	11 (5%)	6 (3%)	5 (8%)	
	Never	191 (80%)	141 (79%)	50 (83%)	
Unprotected Sex While HIV+	Cumulative (Lifetime)	29 (12%)	29 (16%)	0	p = .001
	In the Last Month	13 (5%)	13 (7%)	0	
	In the Last Year	7 (3%)	7 (4%)	0	
	At Least Once	9 (4%)	9 (5%)	0	
	Never	214 (88%)	154 (84%)	60 (100%)	
Unprotected Sex with Someone HIV+	Cumulative (Lifetime)	23 (9%)	23 (12%)	0	p < .01
	In the Last Month	8 (8%)	8 (6%)	0	
	In the Last Year	6 (2%)	6 (3%)	0	
	At Least Once	9 (4%)	9 (5%)	0	
	Never	223 (91%)	163 (88%)	60 (100%)	
Shared Uncleaned FTM Prosthetic Device/ Sex Toy	Cumulative (Lifetime)	14 (6%)	7 (4%)	7 (12%)	p < .05
	In the Last Month	5 (2%)	2 (1%)	3 (5%)	
	In the Last Year	5 (2%)	3 (2%)	2 (3%)	
	At Least Once	4 (2%)	2 (1%)	2 (3%)	
	Never	227 (94%)	175 (96%)	52 (88%)	
Shared Uncleaned Needle(s) for Injection	Cumulative (Lifetime)	9 (4%)	7 (4%)	2 (3%)	N.S.
	In the Last Month	0	0	0	
	In the Last Year	2 (1%)	2 (1%)	0	
	At Least Once	7 (3%)	5 (3%)	2 (3%)	
	Never	232 (96%)	174 (96%)	58 (97%)	

TABLE 6. Bivariate Factors Significantly Associated with HIV+ Status

RISK FACTORS AMONG HIV+ PARTICIPANTS	OTHER	P VALUE
Physical sex at birth Natal Male (97%)	Natal Females (3%)	p < .001
Substance abuse problem (71%)	No substance abuse problem (29%)	p < .001
Sexual assault (27%)	No sexual assault (73%)	p < .001
Unemployment (65%)	Employed (35%)	p < .001
Income < $15k/year (89%)	Income > 15K/year (11%)	p < .001
Violence/crime victimization (68%)	No victimization (32%)	p < .001
Unprotected genital-anal contact ever (87%)	No unprotected G2A contact (13%)	p < .001
Unprotected genital-genital contact ever (93%)	No unprotected G2G contact (7%)	p < .001
Unprotected sex with someone HIV+ ever (28%)	No unprotected sex with someone HIV+ (72%)	p < .001
Unprotected sex while self HIV+ ever (44%)	No unprotected sex while self HIV+ (66%)	p < .001
Sharing uncleaned needles ever (13%)	No sharing uncleaned needles (87%)	p < .001
History of sex work (35%)	No history of sex work (66%)	p < .001
Not having own living space (34%)	Having own living space (66%)	p < .001
Unprotected oral to genital contact ever (90%)	No unprotected O2G contact (10%)	p < .01
Transgender gender identity (84%)	All other gender identities (16%)	p < .01
Job loss due to TG discrimination (26%)	No job loss (74%)	p < .05
African-American race (82%)	All other races (18%)	p < .05
Unprotected manual to genital contact (88%)	No unprotected M2G contact (12%)	p < .05
Had sex while inebriated (61%)	No sex while inebriated (39%)	p < .05

TABLE 7. Logistic Regression Factors Significantly Associated with HIV+ Status

RISK FACTORS AMONG HIV+ PARTICIPANTS	ODDS RATIO	95% CONFIDENCE INTERVAL
Physical sex at birth Female	1	
Natal Males	14.4*	3.0, 70.0
Other race	1	
African-American race	2.5	0.7, 9.1
Other gender identity	1	
Transgender gender identity	1.3	0.4, 3.8
Employed	1	
Unemployed	2.5**	1.1, 5.9
No job loss to discrimination	1	
Lost job to discrimination	1.2	0.4, 3.8
No substance abuse problem	1	
Substance abuse problem	2.2	1.0, 5.1
No sex work	1	
History of sex work	2.8**	1.1, 7.1
No violence/crime victimization	1	
Violence/crime victimization	2.0	0.9, 4.8
No sexual assault	1	
Sexual assault	4.7**	1.3, 16.8

*p < .001, **p < .05

HIV/AIDS related care services as a most important immediate need (48% vs. 33%, p < .05).

DISCUSSION

Sociodemographics

African-Americans were 63% of the total 1997 population of the District of Columbia,[2] versus 70% of the total sample. In this sample, 81% of those reporting their HIV status as positive were African-American. African-Americans were the most likely among the races in our sample to identify their gender identity as transgender (77%, p < .001).

Latino-American participants were over-represented, comprising 22% of the sample, compared to being 7% percent of the 1997 population in the District. However, the official census figures may be low due to the considerable number of undocumented Latinos in the city (in our sample, nearly 7% of the Latino participants lacked residency documents). The

TABLE 8. Demand for Transgender-Specific and Transgender-Sensitive Services

RANK	SERVICE	ALL	NATAL MALES	NATAL FEMALES	P VALUES
1	Transgender-specific HIV education and prevention materials	198 (80%)	153 (82%)	45 (75%)	
2	Transgender-related health care information	194 (78%)	153 (83%)	41 (68%)	p < .05
3	Condom distribution by transgender outreach workers	166 (67%)	126 (67%)	40 (67%)	
4	Transgender-led safer sex seminars	162 (65%)	123 (65%)	39 (65%)	
5	Transgender-specific resource and referral information	152 (61%)	121 (64%)	31 (52%)	
6	Transgender-related hormone prescriptions	147 (59%)	128 (68%)	19 (32%)	p < .001
7	Transgender-sensitive HIV/AIDS testing	126 (51%)	98 (52%)	28 (46%)	
8	Transgender-sensitive case management services	106 (43%)	102 (54%)	4 (7%)	p < .001
9	Vocational training	99 (40%)	94 (50%)	5 (8%)	p < .001
10	Transgender-sensitive legal services	99 (40%)	94 (45%)	15 (25%)	p < .01
11	Transgender-sensitive substance abuse treatment services	92 (37%)	86 (46%)	6 (10%)	p < .001
12	Transgender-staffed hotline/crisis intervention services	90 (36%)	81 (43%)	9 (15%)	p < .001
13	Transportation assistance	76 (31%)	74 (39%)	2 (3%)	p < .001
14	Transgender-related information in native language	32 (13%)	32 (17%)	0	p < .01

TABLE 9. Most Important and Immediate Needs

MOST IMPORTANT IMMEDIATE NEED	ALL	NATAL MALES	NATAL FEMALES	P VALUES
Employment	173 (73%)	132 (74%)	41 (71%)	
Housing	155 (65%)	119 (67%)	36 (62%)	
Job training	125 (53%)	96 (54%)	29 (50%)	
HIV/AIDS-related care services	104 (44%)	85 (48%)	19 (33%)	p < .05
Transgender-related care services	78 (33%)	60 (34%)	18 (31%)	
Routine health care services	54 (23%)	38 (21%)	16 (28%)	

smaller percentage of white participants captured in the sample was probably due to their more closeted nature, their unwillingness to participate possibly due to privacy concerns, and there being fewer of them in a largely African-American city.

The participants were significantly more likely to be natal males rather than females. Male-born participants outnumbered female-born participants at a rate of three-to-one, which corresponds to the estimated prevalence of natal sex for Gender Identity Disorder in the Diagnostic and Statistical Manual of the American Psychiatric Association.[19]

While 65% of all participants (and 79% of the natal males) self-reported their sexual orientation as gay, this data must be carefully interpreted. While transsexual people usually identify their sexual orientation based upon their gender identities, this is not always the case among non-transsexual transgendered people. Other data in the survey suggest that the principal sex partners of the natal male participants were mostly non-transgendered men, and not non-transgendered women, nor other transgendered natal males. Thus, a self-reported gay sexual orientation is understood here as the expression of a desire to identify within cultural or peer group norms, connecting with the larger African-American and Latino gay community, based upon affinity needs or as an expression of solidarity.

In addition to racial and class disparities, the participants' low levels of employment and income may be attributed to the negative impact of discrimination-related factors on educational and employment opportunities. Natal males were more likely to report job loss from discrimination and to lack of health insurance than natal females, possibly due to unemployment or underemployment.

The sample contained high numbers of younger participants, with nearly 80% aged 36 years or less. A possible reason for the high number of youth and young adult participants is that older transgendered people tend to be more closeted and thus less willing to participate in surveys of this kind. However, there is sufficient anecdotal evidence suggesting an undocumented high mortality rate for transgendered residents in the District. Earline Budd, a co-author of this article, has personally made the funeral arrangements for an average of twenty African-American transgendered women who died each year from 1996-2000, many in their youth.

Access to Health Care

Access to regular health care services indicated low levels of regular preventive care (annual physical exams, routine medical screening and gynecological care) among participants. This may be related to their lack of general health care knowledge, but is most likely a result of the participants' low levels of employment and associated lack of health insurance. In the natal anatomy inventory, the participants markedly under-reported their internal anatomical anatomy. While this might be due to issues around their acceptance of possessing this natal anatomy, it is more likely due to a lack of knowledge regarding it. The altered anatomy inventory demonstrated very limited access to surgical sex reassignment procedures.

While significant numbers of participants had accessed transgender-related psychotherapy and hormones, it is quite likely their overall poverty issues removed surgical access from any practical consideration. It also is possible that many participants were either uninformed about or not interested in accessing surgical or cosmetic procedures. Lack of interest in surgical access might therefore be a reflection of the transgender, rather than transsexual, nature of this sample. These findings suggest a need for more health education, not only about surgical options, but also about anatomy and general health care.

Although hormonal therapy was clearly the most sought-after transgender-related medical service, we found it disturbing that 72% of those taking hormones at the time of the survey acquired them on the street. Equally disturbing is that 25% of the natal males had received silicone injections in lieu of hormones, which compares to 30% found in studies conducted in Chicago[20] and New York,[21] and 33% in Los Angeles.[22] Injection Silicone Use and medically unsupervised, self-administration of hormones pose serious risks to the health of transgender people. Street hormone use and Injection Silicone Use may be understandable due to the lack of safer, affordable, alternative means of body modification. At the time of the study, Washington, DC, unlike other major U.S. cities, lacked a clinical program to provide transgender hormonal therapy.

Finally, with the exception of the few participants who accessed sex reassignment surgery, the HBIGDA *Standards of Care (SOC)* were not a significant factor in the participants' access to transgender care. Only 9% of the participants and just over half of their transgender care providers reported knowing about the *SOC*. It is likely that the participants' low incomes, unemployment, and lack of insurance left them unable to simultaneously access psychotherapy, hormonal therapy and surgery, as suggested by the *SOC*.[18] The absence of public funding of these transgender-related services make use of the *SOC* infeasible for most of the participants in our sample.

As a result, participants accessed hormones by other means, either on the streets or from ill-informed doctors who were not regularly measuring liver function and blood levels of hormones. Some natal males engaged in Injection Silicone Use for body modification, either alone or in combination with street hormones. In the assessment of demand for transgender-specific services, the natal males were more likely than natal females to indicate the need to access hormone prescriptions and endocrinology, demonstrating their willingness to access a local clinical transgender hormonal therapy program, if it were available.

Identification of Most Immediate Needs

Overall, the participants cited employment, housing and job training as their three most immediate, important needs. Lack of employment deprived many participants of health insurance and was likely a result of lower educational levels, possibly due to difficult experiences in school. Lack of employment was cited as the principal barrier to housing (by over one-third) but other participants reported the hostility and insensitivity of housing staff and other residents as reasons for their lack of housing.

Suicidal Ideation and Attempts

Studies of transgender populations in other U.S. cities have shown levels of reported suicidal ideation as high as 64% and suicide attempts ranging from 26% to 39%, with most attributing their ideation or attempts to their gender identity issues.[20,23,24,25] In this sample, lower rates of suicidal ideation (38%) and attempts (16%) were found compared to these other studies, perhaps due to the sizeable numbers of African-Americans (70% of all participants) who were least likely among all races in our study to report suicidal ideation. It is interesting that natal females were more likely to report suicidal ideation than natal males, but natal males were more likely to attribute their suicidal ideation to their gender issues. Also notable is that the rate of suicidal ideation in youth (ages 13-19) was high, with the rates dropping significantly in those aged 20-29, then increasing again in those aged 30 and above. It's possible that these youth struggle with their gender identities, then come to terms with many of the issues in their twenties, only to be struck again by the realities of stigmatization and prejudice as they age and work at pursuing careers and family relationships.

Substance Abuse

In other studies,[3,10,11,21,22,26,27,28,29,30] significant substance abuse has been found among transgendered samples, often associated with sex work. Nearly half this sample reported a substance abuse problem, and only half of those reporting substance abuse had ever sought treatment. However, only a third of those with alcohol problems and one-half of those with drug problems sought treatment for them. These findings indicate a need for further study to assess the barriers to accessing treatment when transgendered people acknowledge a substance abuse problem.

HIV Status and Risks

Findings from other studies have reported HIV prevalence in MTF transgendered people as ranging from 14% in San Juan,[29] 19% in Philadelphia,[31] 21% in Chicago,[20] 22% in Los Angeles,[22] 21% to 30% in New York,[21] and 26%,[30] 35%[24] and 47%[28] in San Francisco. Transgender sex workers are at particularly high risk, since they are often financially induced to engage in barrier-free sex.[11,21,28,30] In a study of transgendered sex workers in Atlanta, a 68% seroprevalence rate was reported.[10]

In this sample, we found an overall HIV prevalence rate of 25%, with 32% in natal males. In comparison with other at risk groups ranked by the DC Department of Health in its three year prevention plan,[2] transgendered natal males (MTFs) comprise the group at highest risk in the District of Columbia. HIV status in this sample was self-reported and could not be tested due to cost limitations. If these rates are questionable, however, they likely err on the low side, due to the stigma of disclosing an HIV positive status and the unknown status of those that have not been tested. As in other studies,[20,31] natal males were more likely to get tested than natal females, perhaps due to the higher frequency of their sexual activities.

The most significant factors associated with HIV positive status were being born male, being a victim of sexual assault, having a history of substance abuse and a lack of employment. Interestingly, neither sexual orientation nor level of education were associated with HIV positive status, nor were suicidal ideation and suicide attempts. Among the sexual risk behaviors, unprotected oral to anal contact, unprotected fisting and sharing uncleaned FTM prosthetic devices/dildos were not associated with HIV positive status. Sex reassignment surgery was not significantly associated with HIV negative status, but 10 of the 11 post-operative participants were HIV negative. Hormone use was not associated with HIV status, either with or without doctor monitoring blood hormone levels, or by participants getting hormones on streets. The 3% (n = 2) seroprevalence rate in the natal females of this sample compares with the 2% found in San Francisco.[24] Fifty-three percent of the sample reported being HIV negative, and another 22% did not know their status.

Most alarming were the high levels of unprotected sex reported, identifying a population at a significantly high, immediate risk for HIV/ AIDS and other STDs.

RECOMMENDATIONS

Vocational Training. Employment and job training ranked first and third, respectively, among the most immediate needs of the participants. This suggests that a majority of unemployed participants wished to work, and even those employed sought to better their skills. Development of a pilot program for this population within the District's vocational rehabilitation agency, coupled with transgender sensitivity training for its staff, should be made a priority.

Housing. Housing was the second-most immediate need for participants in the study, directly related to unemployment and underemployment. The lack of affordable housing is an intractable problem that affects many other residents of the District, and does not lend itself to easy solutions. Some possibilities to explore include the establishment in shelters and transitional living houses of transgender-only units or floors; separate rest room facilities if warranted; additional training for staff of assisted housing agencies; and transgender sensitivity programs for non-transgendered residents.

Local Clinical Program for Hormonal Therapy. The inability to pay for transgender-related care; the lack of providers, especially those who are knowledgeable about the blood tests required to avoid complications; the use of street hormones and silicone injections; and high demand all indicate that the implementation of a clinical program in hormonal therapy for transgender residents of the District would be most appropriate. The data regarding the sample's high risks of substance abuse, suicide, Injection Silicone Use and illicit hormone use all suggest an application of the General Theory of Risk Reduction in Transgender Populations, a theory being developed by our coauthor, Ben Singer. The General Theory is based upon the simple premise that people who are happier in their bodies tend to take better care of them.

Studies of HIV, substance abuse and suicide prevention in other populations have identified self-esteem as a key issue in at risk individuals and groups.[32,33,34,35] A probable source of low self-esteem in many transgendered people is their inability to achieve congruence between their physical sex and their internal gender identities. Achievement of this congruence usually includes a passing appearance, allowing many to avoid the associated social stigma. Affording them a medically safe means of body transformation would improve their self-esteem and bodily comfort, producing bodies worth protecting. Anticipated risk reduction would include a lower likelihood of engaging in street hormone use, Injection Silicone Use and substance abuse, and a greater likelihood of practicing safer sex.

A local transgender health program, using hormonal therapy as a magnet, could also offer routine medical screening, not only for HIV and other STDs, but also for cancer, high blood pressure, heart disease and other systemic illnesses. Over time, this risk reduction approach would lower morbidity and mortality rates and greatly improve the health and well-being of transgender residents of the District.

Educational Programs for Transgendered People About Transgender Care. Transgender-related health care information was ranked second highest amongst transgender-specific service needs. Education would empower transgendered people to become informed consumers of transgender-related care. Participants demonstrated a lack of knowledge in several key areas of their own health, specifically in their apparent lack of knowledge of internal reproductive anatomy, the HBIGDA Standards of Care, and the risks of Injection Silicone Use. Peer-led educational programs, working with medical and mental health care providers experienced in dealing with transgendered clients, would be highly beneficial.

Educational Programs for Medical and Mental Health Caregivers About Transgender Care. The data indicated a demonstrable need for better transgender care through more informed providers. Providers of hormonal therapy to many participants were not monitoring their patients' blood chemistries, and lacked knowledge of the HBIGDA *SOC*. Efforts should be made to educate medical providers, beginning at the medical and nursing school levels, followed up by yearly in-service seminars as part of Continuing Medical Education. However, widespread educational efforts in medical and nursing schools would necessarily have to be preceded by successful national advocacy in the U.S. for the acceptance of transgender health care as medically necessary and covered health care benefit. This would require organizations like HBIGDA to assume a public-advocacy role with U.S. public health care agencies and the Congress.

Transgender Sensitivity and Awareness Programs. Although poverty and the lack of health insurance accounted for most of the low overall access of regular medical and transgender care services, provider insensitivity or hostility to transgendered people and a fear of disclosure of transgender status were also commonly reported barriers. Thus in-service trainings about transgendered people, their needs, issues and concerns should be made a permanent part of the required continuing education curricula for professional and service staff members of AIDS Service Organizations, hospitals and other health care delivery facilities, community-based social service organizations, substance abuse treatment facilities, and housing agencies.

Development of Transgender-Specific HIV/ AIDS Education and Prevention Materials. The development of HIV education and prevention specifically targeted at transgendered people is an immediate and pressing need. It was the single most frequently-requested transgender-specific service identified in this assessment (by 80% of all participants). As with other populations, the materials must be culturally-appropriate and sensitive to transgender populations if they are to be effective.

Expansion of Transgender Outreach Efforts. Condom distribution and information about HIV and other STDs by transgender outreach workers ranked third in the transgender-specific services assessment. Expansion of outreach efforts to include additional transgender subpopulations, especially Latino and FTM groups, should be carefully evaluated and implemented.

Additional Research

Further research is urgently needed to develop transgender-specific interventions to halt the spread of HIV infection in this high-risk population.

REFERENCES

1. Centers for Disease Control and Prevention (2002). HIV/AIDS Surveillance Report, Mid-year 2001 Edition, 13(1), February 22, 2002. Atlanta, GA: CDC, http://www.cdc.gov/hiv/stats/hasr1301/. Table 2. AIDS cases and annual rates per 100,000 population, by area and age group, reported through June 2001, United States, available online at: http://www.cdc.gov/hiv/stats/hasr1301/table2.htm.

2. Administration for HIV/AIDS, District of Columbia Department of Health, and The HIV Prevention Community Planning Committee (1999). *District of Columbia HIV Prevention Three Year Plan, 1999-2002.* Administration for HIV/AIDS, District of Columbia Government.

3. Mason, T., Connors, M., & Kammerer, C. (1995). *Transgenders and HIV risks: Needs assessment.* Boston: Gender Identity Support Services for Transgenders.

4. Bockting, W. O., Robinson, B. E., & Rosser, B. R. S. (1998). Transgender HIV prevention: A qualitative needs assessment. *AIDS Care,* 10(4), 505-526.

5. Clements K., Wilkinson W., Kitano K., Ph.D., Marx R., Ph.D. (1999). HIV Prevention and Health Service Needs of the Transgender Community in San Francisco. *International Journal of Transgenderism,* 3, 1&2, and available online at http://www.symposion.com/ijt/hiv_risk/clements.htm.

6. American Public Health Association (2000). APHA Policy Statement 9933: the need for acknowledging transgendered individuals within research and clinical practice. *American Journal of Public Health,* 90: 483-484.

7. Gay and Lesbian Medical Association (2001). *Healthy People 2010 Companion Document for Lesbian, Gay, Bisexual, and Transgender (LGBT) Health* (2001). Gay and Lesbian Medical Association, San Francisco, CA.

8. Green, Jamison (1994). *Investigation into Discrimination Against Transgendered People.* A Report by the Human Rights Commission, City and County of San Francisco, September, 1994. Available online at http://www.ci.sf.ca.us/humanrights/lg_info.html.

9. Claire Skiffington, San Francisco Department of Health, personal communication.

10. Elifson, K., Boles, J., Posey, E., Sweat, M., Darrow, W., and Elsea, W. (1993). Male Transvestite Prostitutes and HIV Risk. *American Journal of Public Health,* 83 (2) 260-262.

11. Boles, J., Elifson, K. (1994). The social organization of transvestite prostitution and AIDS. *Social Science and Medicine*, 39: 85-93.

12. Gender Education & Advocacy, Inc., Remembering Our Dead, http://www.gender.org/remember/.

13. The New York City Gay and Lesbian Anti-Violence Project. *Anti-Lesbian, Gay, Bisexual and Transgender Violence in 1997: A Report of the National Coalition of Anti-Violence Programs*. 1997: The New York City Gay and Lesbian Anti-Violence Project, NY.

14. Castello-Branco, L., Carvalho, M., Castilho, E., Pereira, H., Pereira, M., Galvao-Castro, B. (1988). Frequency of antibody to human immunodeficiency virus (HIV) in male and female prostitutes in Rio de Janeiro, Brazil. Presented at the Fourth International Conference on AIDS, Stockholm, Sweden, June, 1988.

15. Gattari, P., Rezza, G., Zaccarelli, M., Valenzi, C., and Tirelli, U. (1991). HIV infection in drug using transvestites and transsexuals. Letter to the editor, *European Journal of Epidemiology*, 7: 711-712.

16. Modan, B., Goldschmidt, R., Rubenstein, E., Vonsover, A., Zinn, M., Golan, R., Chetrit, A., and Gottlieb-Stematzky, T. (1992). Prevalence of HIV antibodies in transsexual and female prostitutes. *American Journal of Public Health*, 82(4), 590-592.

17. Xavier, J. (2000). *Final report of the Washington Transgender Needs Assessment Survey*, Washington, DC: Administration for HIV and AIDS, Government of the District of Columbia. Available online at http://www.gender.org/resources/dge/gea01011.pdf.

18. Harry Benjamin International Gender Dysphoria Association (2001). *The Standards of Care for Gender Identity Disorders–Sixth Version*, as published in the *International Journal of Transgenderism*, Volume 5, Number 1, January-March 2001, and available online at http://www.symposion.com/ijt/soc_2001/index.htm.

19. American Psychiatric Association (1994). *Diagnostic and Statistical Manual of Mental Disorders, Fourth Edition (DSM IV)*. American Psychiatric Association, Washington, DC.

20. Kenagy, G., & Bostwick, W. (2001). *Health and social service needs of transgendered people in Chicago*. Chicago: Jane Addams College of Social Work, University of Illinois at Chicago.

21. McGowan, C. K. (1999). *Transgender Needs Assessment*. The HIV Prevention Planning Unit of The New York City Department of Health, New York, NY.

22. Reback, C., Simon, P., Bemis, C., & Gatson, B. (2001). *The Los Angeles Transgender Health Study: Community Report*. Los Angeles: University of California at Los Angeles.

23. ActionAIDS, Inc., Unity, Inc., & University of Pennsylvania School of Social Work (1997). *Needs assessment of transgendered people in Philadelphia for HIV/AIDS and other health and social services*. Philadelphia: ActionAIDS, Inc.

24. Clements-Nolle, K., Marx, R., Guzman, R., & Katz, M. (2001). HIV prevalence, risk behaviors, health care use, and mental health status of transgender persons: Implications for public health intervention. *American Journal of Public Health*, 91(6), 915-921.

25. Singer, T. B., Cochran, M., Adamec R. (1997). *Final Report by the Transgender Health Action Coalition (THAC) to the Philadelphia Foundation Legacy Fund* (for the) *Needs Assessment Survey Project* (A.K.A. the Delaware Valley Transgender Survey). Transgender Health Action Coalition: Philadelphia, PA.

26. Reback, C., & Lombardi, E. (1999). HIV risk behaviors of male-to-female transgenders in a community-based harm reduction program. *International Journal of Transgenderism*, 3, 1&2, and available online at http://www.symposion.com/ijt/HIV_risk/reback.htm.

27. Clements, K. et al., *The Transgender Community Health Project: Descriptive Results*. (1999). San Francisco Department of Public Health. Available online at http://hivinsite.ucsf.edu/InSite.jsp?page=kbr-07-04-16&doc=2098.461e.

28. Nemoto, T., Luke, D., Mamo, L., Ching, A., Patria J. (1999). HIV Risk Behaviors Among Male-to-Female Transgenders in Comparison with Homosexual or Bisexual Males and Heterosexual Females. *AIDS Care*, Vol. 11, No. 3, 297-312.

29. Rodríquez-Madera, S. and Toro-Alfonso, J. (2000). Transgenders, HIV and Puerto Rico. Abstract presented at the 2000 United States Conference on AIDS, Atlanta, GA.

30. Nemoto, T., Keatley, J., Operario, D., and Soma, T. (2002). Psychosocial Factors affecting HIV Risk Behaviors among Male to Female transgenders in San Francisco. Abstract # WePeE6583, presented at the International AIDS Conference in Barcelona, Spain, July 2002.

31. Kenagy, G. (2002). HIV among transgender people, *AIDS Care*, Vol. 14, No. 1, 127-134.

32. Crawford, I., Allison, K., Zamboni, B., and Soto, T. (2002). The Influence of Dual-Identity Development on the Psychosocial Functioning of African-American Gay and Bisexual Men. *The Journal of Sex Research*, Vol. 39, No. 3, August 2002, 179-189.

33. Huebner, D., Davis, M., Nemeroff, C., and Aiken, L. (2002). The impact of internalized homophobia on HIV preventive interventions. *American Journal of Community Psychology*, June, 2002; 30(3):327-48.

34. Stokes, J., and Peterson, J. (1998) Homophobia, self-esteem, and risk for HIV among African American men who have sex with men. *AIDS Education and Prevention*, June, 1998 10(3): 278-92.

35. Wingood, G., DiClemente, R., Harrington, K. and Davies, S. (2002). Body Image and African American females' sexual health. *Journal of Women's Health and Gender Based Medicine*, 11(5): 433-439.

The Health and Social Service Needs of Transgender People in Philadelphia

Gretchen P. Kenagy, PhD

SUMMARY. Two Philadelphia-based HIV service organizations and a local university collaborated on a study of health and social service needs of transgender people. Transgender people were the primary resource for the development of the needs assessment survey. In this article, the survey development process, including two discussion groups and two focus groups, are described. Findings on barriers to care, violence, perception of public safety and comfort, suicide and health and social service needs are presented. Total sample size was 81, with 49 male-to-female and 32 female-to-male transgender individuals. Most (68%) were African American. About half of the respondents had thought about attempting suicide. High levels of violence were reported, especially among male-to-females. Health and social service needs included job training/work, dental care, health care, legal services, transportation, education and housing. *[Article copies available for a fee from The Haworth Document Delivery Service: 1-800-HAWORTH. E-mail address: <docdelivery@haworthpress.com> Website: <http://www.HaworthPress.com> © 2005 by The Haworth Press, Inc. All rights reserved.]*

KEYWORDS. Transgender, health access, service needs

INTRODUCTION

Through its HIV prevention outreach program targeting male-to-female (MTF) sex workers, a Philadelphia-based HIV social service organization recognized that it was necessary to have a greater understanding of transgender people's needs regarding HIV. Consequently, the organization applied for and received Ryan White CARE funding to conduct a needs assessment of transgender people in Philadelphia. This organization collaborated with another local social service agency, which provided services to female-to-males (FTMs), and a local university to conduct a needs assessment of MTF and FTM transgender people in Philadelphia. The needs assessment study took place between January and August, 1997.

The purpose of this paper is to provide an overview of the survey development process

Gretchen P. Kenagy, PhD, is affiliated with the Jane Addams College of Social Work, University of Illinois at Chicago.

Address correspondence to: Gretchen P. Kenagy, PhD, Jane Addams College of Social Work, 1040 West Harrison Street, Chicago, IL 60607-7134 (E-mail: kenagy@uic.edu).

The author wishes to thank Kevin Conare, Maureen O. Marcenko, Ben Singer, the focus group and discussion group participants, the interviewers, and the survey respondents.

Support for the needs assessment was provided by Ryan White CARE Act Title I funds, grant 97-21536, through the AIDS Activities Coordinating Office, Philadelphia Health Department.

[Haworth co-indexing entry note]: "The Health and Social Service Needs of Transgender People in Philadelphia." Kenagy, Gretchen P. Co-published simultaneously in *International Journal of Transgenderism* (The Haworth Medical Press, an imprint of The Haworth Press, Inc.) Vol. 8, No. 2/3, 2005, pp. 49-56; and: *Transgender Health and HIV Prevention: Needs Assessment Studies from Transgender Communities Across the United States* (ed: Walter Bockting, and Eric Avery) The Haworth Medical Press, an imprint of The Haworth Press, Inc., 2005, pp. 49-56. Single or multiple copies of this article are available for a fee from The Haworth Document Delivery Service [1-800-HAWORTH, 9:00 a.m. - 5:00 p.m. (EST). E-mail address: docdelivery@haworthpress.com].

Available online at http://www.haworthpress.com/web/IJT
doi:10.1300/J485v08n02_05

and present findings from the needs assessment study. Since the study's findings on HIV/AIDS have been reported previously (Kenagy, 2002), data presented here focus on broader health-related issues (access and barriers to health care, violence, public safety, suicide) and corresponding health and social service needs. Results are presented for the entire sample. Differences between MTFs and FTMs are explored.

DEVELOPMENT OF THE SURVEY INSTRUMENT

Transgender people were the primary resource for the development of the needs assessment survey. An existing instrument developed by a local transgender advocacy group was used as a starting point to obtain ideas on content for the needs assessment survey questionnaire. Two focus groups and two discussion groups with transgender people were held to develop the main topics and many of the questions. The needs assessment survey questionnaire was piloted utilizing feedback from the focus and discussion groups.

Focus Groups

Two focus groups were conducted by the author to identify key issues, which should be included in the survey and to develop language that would be appropriate for and sensitive to transgender people. One group was conducted with MTFs (n = 5) and the other one with FTMs (n = 4); each group lasted about two hours. Participants were recruited from transgender support groups of the collaborating agencies. All except one participant were African American. MTFs ranged in age from 29 to 50 and FTMs were aged 19 to 24. In addition to HIV/AIDS related issues, transgender people in these focus groups made it clear that the scope of the needs assessment needed to be broadened to include a range of health and social service needs that had been severely neglected in their community and that pertain to the context of their HIV risk.

Discussion Groups

The purpose of the discussion groups was to provide a forum for transgender people to re-

view drafts of the needs assessment survey questionnaire for relevance, sensitivity, and appropriateness of the language. Two discussion groups were held, one with MTFs (n = 8) and the other with FTMs (n = 12). Participants suggested several changes and additions to the survey instrument.

MTFs suggested adding questions about people's feelings of safety and comfort in public. They believed that many MTFs were harassed verbally and physically on the street, which caused them to be unwilling or unable to go out in public. They were concerned that if other MTFs were not comfortable going out in public that they might be isolated and in addition, they would be unwilling to come to a social service organization for support.

Both discussion groups wanted the question on gender identity to be open-ended. Discussion group participants stated that the proposed categories (e.g., female-to-male transsexual, male-to-female transsexual, crossdresser, transgenderist) were not familiar to everyone and not used in their communities. It was decided that an open-ended question on gender identity would be used in the survey to allow respondents to express themselves in their own words.

Interviewer Training

Three training sessions were held with potential interviewers. The purpose of the training was to: (1) discuss the important role of the interviewer within the context of the study, (2) discuss techniques for effective face-to-face interviewing, and (3) practice interviewing by having the group members pair-off and administer the full needs assessment survey to each other. None of the people who attended the sessions had previous interviewing experience. Each training sessions lasted about two hours. Twenty people completed the interviewer training.

DATA COLLECTION

Snowball sampling was used to obtain a community-based convenience sample of transgender people in Philadelphia. Respondents were read a statement by the interviewer that introduced the survey and described its purpose. Respondents then signed the consent form giving permission to be interviewed. Inclusion criteria asked participants to identify as transgender by answering "yes" to the following question: "According to one definition, being transgendered is the recognition of conflict between gender at birth and present gender identity. According to this definition do you consider yourself to be transgendered?" People who said "yes" were administered the survey.

One issue that came out of the focus groups was that transgender people may not feel comfortable and may even be fearful of discussing their gender identity with non-transgender people; therefore, in order to be sensitive to these concerns, all of the interviewers were transgender. All interviewers were also associated with the two social service agencies either by employment or participation in a transgender support group. An effort was made to have MTFs interview other MTFs and FTMs interview other FTMs to make it easier for respondents to confide in the interviewers. Also, as a means of helping respondents feel as safe and comfortable as possible, the needs assessment survey was administered to respondents in places of their choosing. As a result, interviews were conducted in a variety of settings, including apartments, boarding homes, restaurants, bars, and on the street. The interviews lasted about one hour. Interviewers were paid seven dollars and respondents received ten dollars for their time.

DATA ANALYSIS

Descriptive statistics (frequencies, percentages, means and standard deviations) were reported on the sample characteristics and health and social service questions. Chi-square and t-test were used to explore the differences between MTFs and FTMs.

RESULTS

Sample Characteristics

There were 81 respondents, 49 MTFs and 32 FTMs. Table 1 provides the demographic characteristics of the total sample and for MTFs and FTMs separately. Sixty-eight percent of respondents were African-American, 12 percent were multiracial, 9 percent were biracial and 12 percent were "other" (including Hispanic and white). The average age of the respondents was 28 years (SD = 6.31), ranging from 19 to 57 years of age. The average number of years of schooling among respondents was 11.7 (SD = 1.5). The majority of the sample (63%) had a high school diploma or GED. FTMs reported attending a significantly higher number of years of schooling than MTFs (t(75) = -2.29, p = .025). Over half of the sample (59%) did not have an employer. FTMs were significantly more likely than MTFs to have an employer (χ^2 (1, n = 80) = 3.86, p = .05).

Although respondents were categorized as MTF or FTM, they described their gender identity in a variety of ways. MTFs described themselves as: "female or feminine" (n = 15), "woman" (n = 7), "butch female" (n = 1), "transsexual female" (n = 3), "transsexual" (n = 3), "MTF" (n = 2), "male" (n = 2), and one person each said "pre-op transsexual," "pre-op female," "ambiguous," "between male and female," "identify with both," "not completely comfortable with gender," "don't know," "love me," "good," and "I'm me." FTMs described their gender identity as: "male" (n = 15), "heterosexual" (n = 3), "female" (n = 3), "transgendered man" (n = 2), and one person each said "FTM," "homosexual female," "very good," and "I'm just me."

When asked "Which of the following terms best describes your sexual orientation right now?" 56 percent of respondents identified as homosexual, 28 percent as heterosexual, 11 percent as bisexual and 5 percent as "other" (responses in this category included asexual). There was a significant difference between MTFs and FTMs on sexual orientation (χ^2 (3, n = 79) = 18.44, p = .000). The majority of FTMs, (84%) in contrast to about one-third of MTFs, (35%) identified their sexual orientation as homosexual.

The sexual orientation terms were not defined in the needs assessment survey, so how these FTMs interpreted the term homosexual is not clear. Findings on sexual activities during the past 3 months, however, illustrated that they engaged in a broad range of sexual activities. Among the 27 homosexual-identified

TABLE 1. Sample Characteristics: Total Sample and by Gender Identity

	Total Sample (N = 81)	MTF (n = 49)	FTM (n = 32)
Average age (SD)	28 (6.3)	29.1 (5.5)	25.4 (7.2)
Average highest grade attended (SD)*	11.7 (1.5)	11.5 (1.6)	12.2 (1.0)
Race			
African-American	68	73	60
Bi/multi-racial	21	17	27
Other (includes Hispanic, white)	12	10	13
Have an employer*	41	33	55
Annual income			
Less than $7,500	27	29	21
$7,500-$14,999	29	26	36
$15,000-$19,999	11	10	14
$20,000-$24,999	22	23	21
$25,000 and above	11	13	7
Sexual Orientation***			
Bisexual	12	16	3
Heterosexual	27	37	13
Homosexual	54	35	84
Other	7	12	0

Note. Due to rounding, percentages may not equal 100%.
*p < .05; ***p < .001

FTMs, 28 percent had oral-penis sex, 42 percent had vagina-penis sex, 42 percent had anal-penis sex, 71 percent had oral-anal sex, 88 percent had oral-vagina sex, and 88 percent had vagina-vagina sex. Since none of these respondents had undergone hormonal treatment or sex reassignment surgery, it appears that they were engaging in same-sex and opposite-sex sexual activities. This is an assumption, however, that needs further exploration. For example, it is not clear how FTMs defined "penis" and, thus, whether or not reports of sex involving a penis meant sex with a natal male.

Access and Barriers to Health Care

To study access to health care, respondents were asked: "Do you have a family doctor or a primary care physician?" Over three-fifths (62%) of respondents reported having a family doctor or primary care physician.

Regarding barriers to health and mental health care, respondents were asked: (1) "Have you ever been refused routine medical care by a doctor or a medical caregiver because you are transgendered?" (2) "Have you ever been refused transgendered related medical care (hormonal or surgical treatment) by a doctor or medical caregiver?" (3) "Have you ever been refused counseling because you are transgender?" and (4) "Have you ever been refused counseling for transgender related issues?"

Fourteen percent of the total sample said they had been refused routine medical care because of their transgender identity. Fifteen percent had been refused transgender related medical care (hormonal or surgical treatment) by a doctor or medical caregiver. Seven percent of respondents had been refused counseling because they were transgender. Ten percent had been refused counseling for transgender related issues. Additionally, when asked, "Does being transgendered create a problem for you when you go for a physical?" 18 percent of respondents said "yes."

Perceived Public Safety

The following two questions were asked about perceptions of safety in public and experiences of violence: (1) "Does being transgendered make you feel unsafe in public?" and (2) "Does being transgendered make you feel uncomfortable in public?" Thirty percent of respondents felt unsafe and 19 percent of respondents felt uncomfortable in public. MTFs were significantly more likely than FTMs to say that they felt unsafe (χ^2 (1, n = 81) = 10.41, p = .001) and uncomfortable in public (χ^2 (1, n = 81) = 12.02, p = .001). Forty-three percent of MTFs, compared to 9 percent of FTMs, felt unsafe, and 31 percent of MTFs, compared to 0 percent of FTMs, reported feeling uncomfortable in public.

One-fifth (20%) of respondents answered, "yes" to the question "Is there any reason you could expect to have a shorter than normal life span?" A significant difference (χ^2 (1, n = 74) = 8.96, p = .003) was found between MTFs and FTMs regarding their perceived life expectancy. Thirty-two percent of MTFs (n = 44) as compared to 3 percent of FTMs (n = 1) expected to have a shorter than normal life span. Reasons MTF respondents gave were: HIV/AIDS, being killed/murdered, disease, stress/pressure of being transgendered, and lack of information.

Three questions regarding violence were asked: (1) "Have you ever been forced to have sex?" (2) "Have you ever experienced violence in your home?" and (3) "Have you ever been physically abused?" The majority of respondents said "yes" to each of the questions (54%, 56%, and 51% respectively). MTFs were significantly more likely than FTMs to have been forced to have sex (χ^2 (1, n = 78) = 11.15, p = .001), experienced violence in their homes (χ^2 (1, n = 81) = 6.33, p = .012) and been physically abused (χ^2 (1, N = 81) = 10.00, p = .01).

Suicide

Respondents were asked (1) "Have you ever thought about attempting suicide?" and (2) "Have you ever attempted suicide?" Just under half (48%) of respondents (n = 79) had thought about attempting suicide and about one-fifth (21%) of respondents (n = 77) had attempted suicide.

If respondents answered "yes" to either or both of the questions on suicide, then they were asked, "Was it because you are transgendered?" Thirty-one percent (11 out of 35) said they thought about attempting suicide because they were transgender and 13 percent (4 out of 31) attempted suicide because they were transgender.

Service Needs

In order to assess service needs, survey participants were asked the following in regard to 17 different service categories: "Are there any of the following services that you need but cannot get?" Table 2 illustrates respondents' reported service needs for all 17 services for the entire sample and by gender identity.

Respondents' top six service needs were: job training/work (75%), dental care (72%), health care (72%), legal services (67%), transportation (65%), education (64%) and housing

(64%). All respondents expressed a high level of service needs. FTMs, however, had significantly higher levels of need than MTFs on most services including child care services (χ^2 (1, n = 76) = 34.59, p = .000), family planning (χ^2 (1, n = 73) = 17.92, p = .000), parenting skills (χ^2 (1, n = 74) = 23.17, p = .000), and transportation (χ^2 (1, N = 81) = 18.75, p = .000).

DISCUSSION

Before discussing the implications of the study findings, some limitations of the study should be addressed. First, the results are limited in their generalizability due to the non-probability sampling method employed. Also, although transgender people in the focus groups and discussion groups did not want to label their gender identity using specific gender identity terms, for purposes of this analysis, partici-

TABLE 2. Service Needs: Total Sample and by Gender Identity

Services Needed	Total Sample (N = 81) %	MTF (n = 49) %	FTM (n = 32) %
Child Care***	37	9	75
Counseling*	61	50	78
Dental Care**	72	59	91
Education*	64	55	78
Family Planning***	38	17	66
Health Care*	71	63	84
Housing*	64	55	78
Information/Referral for HIV/AIDS*	50	38	68
Information/Referral for STD**	53	41	72
Job Training/Work**	75	63	94
Legal Services	67	63	72
Parenting Skills***	43	19	75
Transportation***	65	47	94
Treatment/Rehabilitation for Drug Problems	38	32	48
Treatment/Rehabilitation for Alcohol Problems	34	29	41
Welfare Benefits	47	53	38

*p < .05; **p < .01; ***p < .001

pants were grouped into two gender identity categories (MTF and FTM) so that gender differences could be explored. Transgender identity, however, is complex, encompassing a wide spectrum of gender identities and gender expressions (Green, 2000).

Additionally, the sexual orientation findings highlight the difficulty of applying current conceptions of sexual orientation within a transgender context. For example, the FTMs who identified as homosexual reported engaging in vagina-vagina and penis-vagina sex, but it is unclear whether these activities took place with female- or male-identified partners. Research on lesbian sexuality has found that sexual identity is not solely determined by sexual behavior (Norman, Perry, & Stevenson, 1996). While this may also be true for the FTMs in this sample, sexual orientation among transgender people is likely confounded by gender identity. For people whose gender identity and anatomy are not congruent, the reasons for identifying, as a particular sexual orientation, may be unique from other groups and warrants further study.

The integral involvement of transgender people in every step of the research process was critical to a successful collaboration among the research team members. Focus groups and discussion groups are tools that give people a voice in the research process, which is particularly important for transgender people who are often isolated (Namaste, 1999). Similar to Bockting, Rosser and Coleman (2001), the transgender people who were so integrally involved with the focus groups, discussion groups, and data collection, became invested in the study and were able to use their experiences as a platform for community development by educating transgender and non-transgender people alike about transgender identity.

One such opportunity for education came at a meeting with the HIV Commission of the Philadelphia Extended Metropolitan Area (EMA) AIDS Activity Coordinating Office, Philadelphia Department of Public Health in July, 1997. The study findings were presented at the meeting by a panel consisting of members of the research team including some of the interviewers and members of a local transgender advocacy group. The purpose of the meeting was to discuss never before obtained information on health and social service needs, related to HIV/AIDS particularly, of transgender people in Philadelphia. Early in the presentation, however, members of the commission indicated that they were unfamiliar with the term transgender and had never before met transgender people. The transgender panelists used the opportunity to incorporate basic transgender training ("transgender 101") into the presentation.

Overall, respondents experienced high levels of violence (Bowen, 1995; Courvant, 1997; Reback et al., 2001; Wilchins, Lombardi, Priesing, & Malouf, 1997; Xavier, 2000) and had high levels of suicidal ideation and attempted suicide (Clements, Marx, Guzman, Ideda & Katz, 1998; Xavier, 2000). MTFs seemed to be disproportionately affected by violence-related issues. They were significantly more likely than FTMs to feel uncomfortable and unsafe in public and expect a shorter than normal life span. The reasons for this difference may stem, in part, from the outreach effort made to MTF sex workers during sample recruitment. MTF sex workers are in danger of being victims of violent sexual acts, particularly if they are pre-operative. There is anecdotal information of pre-operative MTFs who have been beaten and even killed by clients who found out they were biological males (Wilchins et al., 1997). MTFs were also more likely than FTMs to have been forced to have sex, experienced violence in their homes and been physically abused. Since respondents were not asked when the violence occurred it is difficult to know if targeting MTF sex workers in the sample had an effect on MTFs' responses to the violence-related questions. Additional study of violence against transgender people, including information on when and in what context abuse takes place as well as the type of abuse is needed.

Findings indicated high levels of need for health and social services, especially among FTMs. This difference may be explained by the services available to both groups at the time of the survey. While health and social services targeting transgender people in Philadelphia were scarce, the existing HIV/AIDS prevention services and support groups seemed to focus on the needs of MTFs. Additionally, MTFs in the sample were more likely to have undergone some aspect of transition [e.g., 86% of MTFs had undergone hormonal treatment as compared to none of the FTMs (χ^2 (1, n = 81) = 56.97, p = .000)]. The FTMs who participated in the focus and discussion groups seemed to have only recently become formally involved in transgender issues through the formation of a FTM support group. Due to snowball sampling, it is likely that the interviewers reached out to respondents who they knew and were similar to them. If this is so, then it is likely that many of the FTM respondents may have only recently identified with a transgender identity. Therefore, in addition to the lack of available services for FTMs, recent identification as transgender may have led FTMs to express higher levels of need for health and social services in comparison to MTFs.

The higher levels of need expressed by FTMs for parenting services compared to MTFs were unexpected and the reasons for the gender difference were not clear. A higher percentage of FTMs (27%) than MTFs (14%) were parents, but this does not fully explain why a majority of FTMs needed these services. Perhaps natal women, despite transgender status are more often the primary caretakers of their children. FTMs might have been socialized as females and, thus, internalized the societal expectation that caring for children is primarily the responsibility of females (Zastrow & Kirst-Ashman, 2001). Additionally, none of the FTMs had undergone medical transition, which may explain why they needed family planning services (see Kenagy & Hsieh, in press).

Findings from this study support other research, which found transgender people experience barriers to accessing health care (JSI Research and Training Institute, 2000; Reback, Simon, Bemis, & Gatson, 2001; Xavier, 2000). Language differences among segments of the transgender community appear to be among the present barriers to service access. Since Virginia Prince coined the term transgender in the mid-1970s to define people like herself who cross-lived full time, but who did not want a surgical sex change (Green & Brinkin, 1994), language that represents the diversity of gender identities within the transgender community has continued to develop. The term transgender is now commonly used in the literature as an umbrella term to describe the multitude of people who identify or express their gender in some way other than their birth-assigned gen-

der including transgenderists, drag queens, cross-dressers, intersex persons, and transsexuals (e.g., Bockting et al., 2001). What is unclear, however, is whether or not there is continuity in the interpretation and usage of this language across ethnic sub-groups of transgender people. At the time of this study, respondents, the majority of whom were people of color, described their gender identity in a multitude of ways and did not appear to be using a common set of terms to describe their gender identity. A mismatch of language (Lum, 1999) between health and social service providers and transgender people can result in barriers to services. Organizations serving the transgender community may find it useful to address issues pertaining to ethnicity concomitantly with gender identity to reduce potential barriers for transgender people who are attempting to identify and access services that are appropriate to their needs.

Transgender people may also face geographic barriers to services. As discussed earlier, going out in public may feel uncomfortable or unsafe to some transgender people, particularly MTFs who fear they may be targeted for harassment. This could restrict their ability to access service organizations as they might not feel able or willing to travel very far from their homes and neighborhoods.

It is recommended that organizations increase their outreach to transgender people. Services should be located in places where they live, work and socialize to provide a safe and accessible service environment. Trust in the agency may be heightened by hiring transgender people as part of the outreach team (Kammerer, Mason, Connors, & Durkee, 2001). This would give transgender people valuable employment experience and financial resources, and agencies would more easily develop ties to a hard-to-reach population. Identifying the needs of transgender people and developing programs and services to meet those needs has begun to take place in many major cities across the U.S. As the work continues to move forward, attention must continually be given to the barriers faced by the transgender community, including ethnic minorities, so that all transgender people are afforded needed health and social services.

REFERENCES

Bockting, W. O., Rosser, B. R. S., & Coleman, E. (2001). Transgender HIV prevention: community involvement and empowerment. In W. Bockting & S. Kirk (Eds.), *Transgender and HIV: Risks, prevention, and care* (pp. 119-144). New York: The Haworth Press, Inc.

Bowen, G. (1995). *Violence and health poll.* (Available from The American Boyz, P. O. Box 1118, Elkton, MD, 21922-1118).

Clements, K., Marx, R., Guzman, R., Ikeda, S. & Katz, M. (1998). Prevalence of HIV infection in transgendered individuals in San Francisco. Poster presented at the XII International Conference on AIDS, Geneva, Switzerland.

Courvant, D. (1997). *Domestic violence and the sex- or gender-variant survivor.* (Available from the Survivor Project, 5028 NE 8th, Portland, OR 97211).

Dekker, R. M. & van de Pol, L. C. (1989). *The tradition of female transvestism in early modern Europe.* New York: St. Martin's.

Green, J. (2000). Introduction to transgender issues. In P. Currah, & S. Minter, S. *Transgender equality: A handbook for activists and policymakers* (pp. 1-12). National Gay and Lesbian Task Force. Retrieved December 6, 2003, from *http://www.ngltf.org/library/index.cfm#2.*

Green, J., & Brinkin, L. (1994). *Investigation into discrimination against transgendered people.* Human Rights Commission City and County of San Francisco Report. San Francisco: Human Rights Commission.

Kammerer, N., Mason, T., Connors, M., Durkee, R. (2001). Transgender health and social service needs in the context of HIV risk. In. W. Bockting, & S. Kirk (Eds.). *Transgender and HIV: Risks, prevention, and care* (pp. 39-57). New York: The Haworth Press, Inc.

Kenagy, G. P. (2002). HIV among transgendered people. *AIDS Care, 14,* 127-134.

Kenagy, G. P. & Hsieh, C.M. (In press). Gender differences in the social service needs of transgender people. *Journal of Social Service Research.*

Lum, D. (1999). Culturally competent practice: A framework for growth and action. Pacific Grove, CA: Brooks/Cole Publishing Company.

JSI Research & Training Institute, Inc., (2000). *Access to health care for transgendered persons in greater Boston.* Boston: GLBT Health Access Project.

Namaste, V. K. (1999). HIV/AIDS and female to male transsexuals and transvestites: Results from a needs assessment in Quebec. *International Journal of Transgenderism.* Retrieved March 29, 2002, from *http://www.symposion.com/itj/hiv_risk/namaste.htm.*

Norman, A. D., Perry, M. J., & Stevenson, L. Y. (1996). Lesbian and bisexual women in small cities–At risk for HIV? *Public Health Reports, 111,* 347-352.

Reback, C. J., Simon, P. A., Bemis, C. C., & Gatson, B. (2001). *The Los Angeles transgender health study: Community report.* Los Angeles: Authors.

Wilchins, R. A, Lombardi, E., Priesing, D., & Malouf, D. (1997). *First national survey of transgender violence.* New York: GenderPAC.

Xavier, J. M. (2000). *The Washington transgender needs assessment survey.* Retrieved January 15, 2002, from *http://www.gender.org/vaults/wtnas.html.*

Zastrow, C., & Kirst-Ashman, K. K. (2001). *Understanding human behavior in the social environment.* Belmont, California: Wadsworth.

Health and Social Service Needs
of Transgender People in Chicago

Gretchen P. Kenagy, PhD
Wendy B. Bostwick, MPH

SUMMARY. A needs assessment of transgender people was conducted in Chicago in 2001 to assess their HIV risks, health and social service needs, and barriers to care. One hundred and eleven transgender individuals, 78 male-to-females (MTFs) and 33 female-to-males (FTMs), participated in the study. Fourteen percent of respondents reported being HIV-positive; they were all male-to-female and the majority was of color. Risk factors for HIV included unprotected sex and willingness to have high-risk sex in the future. Respondents experienced high levels of violence. Two-thirds of respondents had thought of attempting suicide. Respondents reported a high need for health and social services, particularly MTFs and people of color. *[Article copies available for a fee from The Haworth Document Delivery Service: 1-800-HAWORTH. E-mail address: <docdelivery@ haworthpress.com> Website: <http://www.HaworthPress.com> © 2005 by The Haworth Press, Inc. All rights reserved.]*

KEYWORDS. Transgender, health, services, barriers

INTRODUCTION

A growing body of literature in the past decade has documented that transgender persons have a wide range of health and service needs (e.g., Bockting, Robinson, & Rosser, 1998; Clements, Marx, Guzman, Ikeda, & Katz, 1998; Kammerer, Mason, & Connors, 1999; Xavier, 2000). Included among the health issues emerging from the literature are violence, suicide, HIV/AIDS and barriers to health care access. Studies to date have found that transgender people are at risk for HIV and AIDS through unprotected anal and vaginal sex and unclean needles, as well as high levels of HIV infection among MTFs (Clements et al., 1998; Elifson et al., 1993; Kenagy, 2002; Reback, Simon, Bemis, & Gatson, 2001).

Violence and suicide are also health-related issues of particular concern to transgender people (Courvant, 1997; Mackenzie, 1994). Research shows that transgender people are

Gretchen P. Kenagy, PhD, and Wendy B. Bostwick, MPH, are both affiliated with the Jane Addams School of Social Work, University of Illinois at Chicago.

Address correspondence to: Gretchen P. Kenagy, PhD, Jane Addams School of Social Work, 1040 West Harrison Street, Chicago, IL 60607-7134 (E-mail: kenagy@uic.edu).

The authors would like to express their appreciation for those who made this study possible. The authors owe many thanks to the respondents for taking time to participate in the study. Their sincere thanks also to the interviewers for their diligence in recruiting and interviewing respondents.

[Haworth co-indexing entry note]: "Health and Social Service Needs of Transgender People in Chicago." Kenagy, Gretchen P., and Wendy B. Bostwick. Co-published simultaneously in *International Journal of Transgenderism* (The Haworth Medical Press, an imprint of The Haworth Press, Inc.) Vol. 8, No. 2/3, 2005, pp. 57-66; and: *Transgender Health and HIV Prevention: Needs Assessment Studies from Transgender Communities Across the United States* (ed: Walter Bockting, and Eric Avery) The Haworth Medical Press, an imprint of The Haworth Press, Inc., 2005, pp. 57-66. Single or multiple copies of this article are available for a fee from The Haworth Document Delivery Service [1-800-HAWORTH, 9:00 a.m. - 5:00 p.m. (EST). E-mail address: docdelivery@haworthpress.com].

subjected to varying forms of violence including physical abuse (Bowen, 1995; Kenagy, 1998; Reback et al., 2001; Wilchins, Lombardi, Priesing, & Malouf, 1997; Xavier, 2000), sexual abuse (Bowen, 1995; Clements et al., 1998; Kenagy, 1998; Wilchins et al., 1997) and verbal abuse (Reback et al., 2001).

In terms of suicide, it has long been speculated that transsexuals are prone to suicide (Block & Tessler, 1973; Levine, 1978; Wicks, 1977), but few empirically based studies of transgender people have included questions on suicide. The information that does exist, however, gives reason for concern about suicide in this population. In San Francisco, 32% (N = 515) of transgender individuals had attempted suicide (Clements et al., 1998). Also, about one-third (30%) of transgender people in Philadelphia (N = 176) attempted suicide; 67% of them did so because they were transgender (Kenagy, in press). The rate of attempted suicide among a sample of 252 in Washington, D.C., was lower at 16% (Xavier, 2000). Over one-third (35%) of these respondents, however, reported suicidal ideation and among them, 64 percent had thought about suicide because of their gender issues (Xavier, 2000).

Another health-related issue facing the transgender community is barriers to care. Studies have found, for example, that transgender people experience discrimination due to their gender identity when trying to obtain or access health and social services (Bowen, 1995; JSI Research and Training Institute, 2000; Reback et al., 2001; Warren, 1999; Xavier, 2000). Reback et al. (2001) found that 244 transgender women (MTFs) in Los Angeles attributed their gender identity and/or presentation as the reason they had difficulties obtaining a job (47%), had lost a job (28%) and were either denied or had lost housing (30%). Among a sample of 392 MTFs and 123 FTMs, in San Francisco, 46 percent of MTFs and 57 percent of FTMs reported job discrimination and 27 percent of MTFs and 21 percent of FTMs reported housing discrimination based on gender identity or gender presentation (Clements et al., 1998). While transgender identity has resulted in outright refusal of services, some organizations have offered their services contingent upon transgender people wearing clothing appropriate to their birth-assigned gender (Kammerer,

Mason, Connors, & Durkee, 2001; Namaste, Laframboise, & Brady, n.d.).

While needs assessment studies have provided important information about the effect of gender identity on access to services, rarely have transgender people been directly asked about their social service needs. Xavier (2000), however, did find high levels of need for housing and employment training among a sample of 252 transgender people, primarily of color, in Washington, D.C.

To fill the gap in empirically-based knowledge about the health and social service needs of transgender people in Chicago, we conducted a needs assessment study from September, 2000 to March, 2001. The survey was the first of its kind in Chicago and was intended to support the local transgender community and provider organizations in the development of health and social services for transgender people in Chicago.

METHODS

The needs assessment study is a replication of a needs assessment in the Philadelphia area (Kenagy, 2002). The study was funded by the University of Illinois at Chicago (UIC) Campus Research Board (CRB) and approved by the UIC Institutional Review Board (IRB).

Procedure

Participants were recruited using snowball sampling. Ten transgender interviewers were trained to conduct structured face-to-face interviews in locations of the respondent's choosing, which included their homes, in restaurants and on the street. Respondents were considered eligible to participate in the study, if they answered "yes" to the following question: "According to one definition, being transgendered is the recognition of conflict between gender at birth and present gender identity. According to this definition, do you consider yourself to be transgendered?" Participants received a $20 cash stipend upon conclusion of the interview.

Instrument/Questions

The survey instrument was developed collaboratively with transgendered people and pilot tested. Focus groups and discussion groups were held with transgender people to develop the main topics and many of the questions for the needs assessment survey. Questions on AIDS knowledge, perceived current and future risk, status and testing were obtained from the National Health Interview Survey, 1992: AIDS Knowledge and Attitudes Supplement (U.S. Department of Health and Human Services, 1993). The following are major variables from the needs assessment survey reported in the results section:

Age. Age, in years, was the respondent's age at interview.

Education. Education was the years of schooling completed.

Race. Respondents were asked to identify their race. Race was categorized as People of color and white.

Employment. Respondents were asked to answer "yes" or "no" to the question "Do you have an employer right now?"

Sexual orientation. Respondents were asked: "Which of the following terms best describes your sexual orientation right now? Heterosexual, Homosexual, Bisexual, Asexual, Other, Don't know."

AIDS knowledge. Respondents were read 11 statements about AIDS and given a choice of answering "true," "false," or "don't know." Respondents' AIDS knowledge score was based on the number of correctly answered questions.

Perceived susceptibility to AIDS. Respondents were asked two questions about their perceived current and future risk for AIDS: (1) "What are your chances of *having* the AIDS virus; would you say high, medium, low or none?" and (2) "What are your chances of *getting* the AIDS virus; would you say high, medium, low or none?"

Current HIV risk. Respondents were considered to be at current risk for HIV infection if they engaged in one or more of the following activities without using a latex barrier such as a dental dam or a condom during the three months prior to the interview: vagina-penis, anal-penis, oral-penis, oral-vagina, oral-anal or vagina-vagina sex. In addition, they were considered to be at risk if they had sex while drunk or high or had sex with someone known to be HIV-positive during the three months prior to the interview.

Future HIV risk. Respondents were also asked about their willingness to engage in one or more of the following in the future: sex without a latex barrier such as a condom or dental dam, sex with multiple partners at the same time or non-monogamous sex, sex while drunk or high, or sex with someone who was known to be HIV-positive.

HIV testing. Respondents were asked "(Except for blood donations since March 1985) have you had your blood tested for the AIDS virus infection?" Respondents who said they had been tested were asked "How long ago was your most recent test?" Answers were recorded in months.

HIV status. Respondents were asked to answer "yes" or "no" to the question "As far as you know, are you HIV positive?"

STD testing. Respondents were asked "Have you ever been tested for a sexually transmitted disease (STD) other than HIV/AIDS?" Respondents who said they had been tested were asked "How long ago was your most recent test?" Answers were recorded in months.

STD status. Respondents were asked to answer "yes" or "no" to the question "As far as you know, have you ever had an STD?"

Drug and needle use. Respondents were asked "Have you ever injected any drugs?" Respondents who reported injecting drugs were asked: "Do you think you have ever used a needle that wasn't new and clean?" Respondents were also asked whether or not they thought the needles they used for hormonal treatment, silicone injections, electrolysis and tattooing were clean.

Hormone use. Respondents were asked "Have you ever obtained hormones from a source other than a licensed physician?"

Perceived public safety. Respondents were asked to answer "yes" or "no" to the questions (1) "Does being transgendered make you feel unsafe in public?" (2) "Does being transgender made you feel uncomfortable in public?" and (3) "Is there any reason you could expect to have a shorter than normal life span?"

Violence. Respondents were asked to answer "yes" or "no" to the questions (1) "Have you ever been forced to have sex?" (2) "Have you ever experienced violence in your home?" and (3) "Have you ever been physically abused?"

Suicide. Respondents were asked "Have you ever thought about attempting suicide?" and "Have you ever attempted suicide?" If respondents answered "yes" to either question, the follow-up question "Was it because you are transgendered?" was asked.

Health access and barriers. Respondents were asked ten questions regarding access and barriers to medical and mental health care services. (1) Do you have a family doctor or a primary care physician? (2) Do you have health insurance? (3) Have you ever been refused routine medical care by a doctor or a medical caregiver because you are transgendered? (4) Have you ever been refused transgendered-related medical care (hormonal or surgical treatment) by a doctor or medical caregiver? (5) Have you ever had difficulty getting emergency health care because you are transgendered? (6) Does being transgendered create a problem for you when you go for a physical? (7) Do you have anyone you can talk to about transgender-related issues? (8) Have you ever gone to a counselor for help in dealing with transgender-related issues? (9) Have you ever been refused counseling for transgender related issues? (10) Have you ever been refused counseling because you were transgender?

Service needs. Respondents were given a list of sixteen services: transportation, housing, job training, education, child care, family planning, parenting skills, counseling, health care, dental care, legal services, STD information/referral, HIV information/referral, treatment/rehabilitation for drug problems, treatment/rehabilitation for alcohol problems, and welfare benefits. This list of services came out of discussions with transgender people during focus groups that took place during the development of the needs assessment survey questionnaire.

Analysis

Results are presented for the entire sample. Differences between MTFs and FTMs, as well as people of color and whites, are explored using T-test and Chi-square. Given the exploratory nature of the study and multiple comparisons, a p value of .01 has been set to determine statistical significance.

RESULTS

Participants

Of the 111 respondents, 70% (n = 78) were male-to-female (MTF) and 30% (n = 33) were female-to-male (FTM). Table 1 provides the demographic characteristics of the total sample and for MTFs and FTMs separately. The sample was 43% white, 34% African-American and 23% biracial, multiracial or "other" (including Asian, Native American, Hispanic). When the two racial groupings were created, there were 60 people of color and 51 whites. Note that the Hispanic non-black respondents (n = 3) were coded as white.

The average age of respondents (n = 108) was 35 years (SD = 11.9), ranging from 19 to 70 years of age. The majority of respondents (62%) had at least some college education and two-thirds of the sample (66%) reported that they had an employer. Thirty percent of respondents identified as heterosexual, 26% as other, 24% as homosexual, 14% as bisexual, and 7% as asexual. A significant difference in sexual orientation was found between MTFs and FTMs, χ^2 (4, n = 101) = 28.73, p = .000. Thirty-nine percent of MTFs identified as heterosexual as compared to 7 percent of FTMs and 57 percent of FTMs identified their sexual orientation as "other," compared to 13 percent of MTFs. FTMs who said "other" defined sexual orientation as "queer" (n = 8), "pansexual" (n = 2), "sexual" (n = 1) and "no label" (n = 1).

AIDS Knowledge

The average score of respondents' answers to eleven AIDS knowledge questions was 10.10 (SD = .999) and ranged from 7 to 11. Regarding perceived AIDS knowledge, over half of respondents (54%) said they knew "a little," 42 percent said "some," and only 4 percent said they knew "a lot" about AIDS.

HIV/AIDS Risk

Among the 86 HIV negative respondents who answered the question, most perceived they had either a low chance (51%) or no chance (37%) of having AIDS. Similarly, among the 62

TABLE 1. Sample Characteristics: Total Sample and by Gender Identity

	Total Sample (N = 111)	MTF (n = 78)	FTM (n = 33)	People of Color (n = 61)	White (n = 50)
Average Age (SD)	34.8 (11.9)	38.3 (11.6)	26.9 (8.3)	33.7 (9.4)	36.0 (14.2)
Average Highest Grade Attended (SD)[a]**	13.9 (2.5)	13.4 (2.7)	14.5 (1.8)	12.7 (2.0)	15.1 (2.3)
	%	%	%	%	%
Gender Identity[a]**					
MTF	70	-	-	83	55
FTM	30	-	-	17	45
Race					
African-American	34	42	9	-	-
Bi/Multi-Racial	13	12	12	-	-
White	43	32	70	-	-
Other (includes Asian, Latino, Native American	10	10	9	-	-
Have an Employer[a]**	66	58	82	51	82
Annual Income					
Less than $10,000	19	18	21	24	13
$10,000-$19,999	21	18	29	20	23
$20,000-$29,999	19	18	21	18	21
$30,000-39,999	13	13	14	16	10
$40,000 and above	27	34	5	22	33
Sexual Orientation[a]**[b]**					
Asexual	7	10	0	5	9
Bisexual	14	17	7	9	20
Heterosexual	30	39	7	46	9
Homosexual	24	21	30	23	24
Other	26	13	57	16	38

Note. Due to rounding, percentages may not equal 100%.
[a] a significant difference between whites and people of color.
[b] a significant difference between MTFs and FTMs.
**p < .001

respondents who answered the question on future AIDS risk, 69% perceived their chances were low and 21% thought they had no chance of getting AIDS.

Three-fifths of respondents (61%) had engaged in at least one unprotected vaginal, anal, or oral sex activity during the three months prior to being interviewed. FTMs were significantly more likely than MTFs to have done so,

χ^2 (1, n = 108) = 14.33, p = .000; about half (49%) of MTFs and most (88%) of FTMs had sex without a latex barrier. Additionally, 41 percent of respondents had engaged in sexual activity while drunk or high and/or with someone they knew was HIV positive. Among those who were HIV positive (15 out of 16 responded), 67 percent had engaged in sex without a latex barrier and 81 percent had engaged in sexual activity while drunk or high and/or with someone they knew was HIV positive.

Seventy-nine percent of respondents indicated that they would engage in one or more high risk sexual activities in the future; the difference between MTFs (71%) and FTMs (97%) was significant, χ^2 (1, N = 111) = 8.95, p = .003. Specifically, FTMs were more likely than MTFs to engage in unprotected sex (94% versus 52%), χ^2 (1, n = 104) = 17.41, p = .000; non-monogamous sex (82% versus 36%), χ^2 (1, n = 105) = 18.91, p = .000; sex while drunk or high (79% versus 40%), χ^2 (1, n = 105) = 13.45, p = .000; and sex with an HIV-positive person (53% versus 18%), χ^2 (1, n = 100) = 13.30, p = .000.

HIV/STD Testing and Status

The majority of respondents (69%) stated that they had been tested for HIV. People of color (78%) were more likely than whites (57%) to have been tested, χ^2 (1, N = 111) = 5.89, p = .015. Among the HIV negative respondents who provided data (n = 58), 64% were tested an average of 20.63 months ago (SD = 30.11, range 1-180). Sixteen respondents (15%) reported being HIV positive. All were MTF and disproportionally people of color (94%), χ^2 (1, n = 106) = 13.23, p = .000.

Most respondents (71%) reported having been tested for an STD, on an average of 38.72 months ago (SD = 66.71, range 1-300). People of color (78%) were more likely than whites (57%) to have been tested, χ^2 (1, N = 111) = 5.89, p = .015. Twenty-two percent of respondents (n = 108) reported having had at least one STD including gonorrhea (n = 8), syphilis (n = 6), chlamydia (n = 3), herpes (n = 2) and pubic lice (n = 1).

Drug and Needle Use

The majority (88%) of the 110 respondents who answered the question on injection drug use had not injected drugs during their lifetimes. Of the 13 respondents who reported injecting drugs, 54% were FTM and 46% had used a needle that wasn't new and clean. Most (90%) of 57 respondents thought the needles were clean for hormone injections as well as silicone injections, (85% of 27 respondents),

electrolysis (94% of 47 respondents), and tattooing (92% of 37 respondents).

Additionally, two-fifths (40%) of respondents reported obtaining hormones from a source other than a licensed physician. MTFs (53%) were more likely than FTMs (9%), χ^2 (1, n = 110) = 18.77, p = .000, and respondents of color (56%) were more likely than whites (22%), χ^2 (1, n = 110) = 13.46, p = .000, to have done so.

Perceived Public Safety

Fifty-six percent of respondents reported that being transgender made them feel unsafe in public and 43 percent reported that being transgender made them feel uncomfortable in public. FTMs were significantly more likely than MTFs to say that they felt unsafe, χ^2 (1, n = 109) = 16.02, p = .000, and uncomfortable in public, χ^2 (1, n = 110) = 17.34, p = .000. Eighty five percent of FTMs compared to 43 percent of MTFs felt unsafe, and 73% of FTMs compared to 30% of MTFs reported feeling uncomfortable in public. In addition, 40% of all respondents felt that their life span may be shorter than normal. Reasons given were queer-bashing, being killed by the police, the effects of hormones and HIV status.

Violence and Suicide

Forty-six percent of respondents reported that they had been forced to have sex, 66% reported violence in the home and 60% said they had been physically abused at some point during their lives.

Sixty-four percent of respondents said that they had thought about attempting suicide. Whites (77%) were more likely than people of color (52%) to report suicidal ideation, χ^2 (1, n = 107) = 7.02, p = .008. Two-thirds (60%) of those who considered suicide and for whom there is data (n = 57) did so because they were transgendered. Twenty-seven percent of respondents (n = 108) reported attempting suicide. Over half (52%) of the 25 people who answered the question said they had attempted suicide because they were transgender.

Health Access and Barriers

Health care. Seventy-two percent of the total sample reported that they had a doctor or primary care physician. Two-thirds of respondents (65%) said that they had health insurance. Whites (80%) were significantly more likely than people of color (52%) to have been insured, χ^2 (1, n = 110) = 9.57, p = .002.

Twelve percent of respondents stated that they had been refused routine medical care because of their transgender identity; 23 percent said they had been refused transgender-related medical care. Fourteen percent reported difficulty getting emergency health care because they were transgender. Finally, 38% of respondents stated that being transgender created a problem for them when going for a physical. This was more likely among FTMs (69%) than MTFs (25%), χ^2 (1, n = 105) = 18.34, p = .000.

Mental health care. Almost all of the respondents (94%) reported having someone to talk to about transgender-related issues. Two-thirds of the sample (66%) had seen a counselor for transgender-related issues. Nine percent said that they had been refused counseling for transgender-related issues and only 3 percent had been refused counseling because they were transgender.

Service Needs

Respondents' top five service needs were: dental care (36%), education (32%), legal services (32%), health care (31%) and job training/work (27%) (see Table 2). MTFs were significantly more likely than FTMs to need transportation, χ^2 (1, n = 109) = 9.36, p = .002, and welfare benefits, χ^2 (1, n = 106) = 5.69, p = .017. Nearly one quarter of MTFs (23%) said that they needed transportation compared to zero FTMs; 23 percent of MTFs stated a need for welfare benefits compared to 3 percent of FTMs.

In addition, there were six categories in which MTFs stated a need for services but none of the FTMs did. These were: child care, family planning, parenting skills, information and referral for HIV/AIDS, and information and re-

TABLE 2. Service Needs: Total Sample and by Gender Identity and Race

Service(s) Needed	Total Sample (N = 111)	MTF (n = 78)	FTM (n = 33)	White (n = 50)	People of Color (n = 61)
	%	%	%	%	%
Child Care	8	12	0	2	14
Counseling	24	24	24	20	28
Dental Care[a*]	36	39	30	22	38
Education	32	36	21	20	42
Family Planning	9	13	0	2	15
Health Care	31	32	27	22	38
Housing[a**]	23	31	6	4	40
Information/Referral for HIV/AIDS	9	13	0	2	15
Information/Referral for STD	10	14	0	2	17
Job Training/Work	27	34	12	14	38
Legal Services[a**]	32	36	21	14	47
Parenting Skills	10	15	0	2	17
Transportation[b**]	16	23	0	8	24
Treatment/Rehabilitation for Drug Problems	7	10	0	2	12
Treatment/Rehabilitation for Alcohol Problems	7	9	3	4	10
Welfare Benefits[a*b**]	17	23	3	4	28

Note. Due to rounding, percentages may not equal 100%.
[a] a significant difference between whites and people of color.
[b] a significant difference between MTFs and FTMs.
*p < .01; **p < .001

ferral for STDs and treatment for drug problems. Both MTFs and FTMs, however, reported similar needs for health care, dental care and counseling.

There were also significant differences among four service needs between whites and people of color. Nearly half (48%) of people of color reported a need for legal services compared to 16% of whites, χ^2 (1, n = 104) = 11.64, p = .001. People of color were more likely than whites to say that they needed housing (40% vs. 4%), χ^2 (1, n = 110) = 19.58, p = .000. People of color also reported a higher need for dental care at 48% compared to 22% of whites, χ^2 (1, N = 111) = 8.57, p = .003, and for welfare benefits at 29% compared to 4% of whites, χ^2 (1, n = 106) = 11.29, p = .001.

DISCUSSION

There are a few limitations in this study that should be considered before discussing the findings. Study participants were recruited using the snowball sampling method, and therefore, results are limited in their generalizability. In addition, the authors recognize that by grouping participants into two discrete gender identity categories, we are in some sense reinforcing the notion of gender as a binary. In reality, of course, transgender identity encompasses a wide spectrum of gender identities and expressions (Green, 2000). Similarly, the racial category "people of color" is made up of many racial/ethnic categories.

Despite the limitations, the findings from this study compliment the literature by reporting the health-related issues as well as the health and social service needs of transgender persons in Chicago. There are a number of significant findings worth noting. First, this study found a high rate of HIV infection among MTFs, which supports findings from previous studies (Clements-Nolle et al., 2001; Kenagy, 2002; Reback et al., 2001; Xavier, 2000). Over one-fifth of MTFs reported that they were HIV positive. In fact, given that these are self-report results and no additional blood tests were conducted, it is likely that this percentage underrepresents HIV prevalence in this sample.

A particularly disturbing finding was that 15 out of the 16 individuals who reported that they were HIV positive were MTFs of color, indicating a significant disparity between whites and people of color in terms of HIV status. This finding reflects the overall picture of HIV infection in the U.S., as people of color and women continue to be disproportionately affected by the disease (National Institute of Allergy and Infectious Diseases, 2002; Centers for Disease Control and Prevention, n.d.). Worth noting, however, is that respondents of color were more likely to report being tested for HIV than their white counterparts. Thus, there is the potential for this disparity, to some degree, to be a reflection of testing bias. Nevertheless, the continued finding of such high-rates of HIV among MTFs, particularly MTFs of color suggests the immediate need for targeted strategies and prevention programs, as well as HIV care services tailored to transgender populations.

Previous studies found FTMs to be at risk for HIV infection from high levels of unprotected sex, willingness to engage in high-risk sexual activities in the future, lack of recent testing for HIV and other STDs (Kenagy, 2002), lack of information about transgender sexuality, lack of access to intramuscular needles, low self esteem (Namaste, 1999) and the belief that they were not at risk for infection (Kenagy, 2002; Namaste, 1999). This study also found FTMs at risk for HIV infection, particularly from high-risk/unprotected sex. Future HIV risk assessments should be FTM inclusive and take into consideration the uniqueness of their bodies (Bockting et al., 1998), as well as their sexual activities so that the exact nature of their risk for HIV as well as other STDs can be understood.

Second, this study found high levels of suicidal ideation and attempted suicide. These findings support data from previous studies that suicide is a major health concern among transgender people (Clements-Nolle et al., 2001; Xavier, 2000). While there is no official national data in the United States for suicide attempt, it is estimated that there are 730,000 suicide attempts in the U.S. each year (American Association of Suicidology, 2001), which is about the rate of .002, or 200 attempts per 100,000 persons. Within this context, the high percentage of reported suicide attempts among the study sample is alarming. Also of concern is the high percentage of respondents in this study who cited being transgender as the reason they thought about attempting suicide (51%) and/or who attempted suicide (46%).

Third, on a positive note, almost all of the respondents had someone to talk with about transgender-related issues. In comparison to medical services, lower rates of counseling service refusal were found, suggesting that mental health care may be more accessible to transgender people than medical care.

Similar to studies by Xavier (2000) and the JSI Research & Training Institute (2000), however, the results of this study indicate that transgender people experienced difficulties in accessing health care services. For example, while two-thirds of the sample had health insurance, respondents of color were significantly less likely to have coverage. This may reflect the fact that people of color were less likely to have an employer. Without employment opportunities, not only is one's ability for self support in jeopardy, but so is access to the health care system. The findings indicate that people of color are not receiving health care through public assistance programs either. While respondents were not directly asked about their use of Medicaid, out of the 20 who reported being on public assistance–most of whom were people of color (16) and MTF (19)–17 were receiving Supplemental Security Income (SSI) or Supplemental Security Disability Income (SSDI). Although most people on these programs are eligible for Medicaid (DiNitto, 2000), only 3 of the respondents on SSI/SSDI, listed Medicaid under the response option "other" (the remaining three respondents on public assistance received food stamps). Therefore, it remains unclear why people of color were having difficulty accessing health insurance and health services. Perhaps, lack of ability to obtain documents such as a drivers license consistent with their present name and gender identity was a contributing factor. Research is needed to further explore health access issues among transgender people, particularly those of color.

Also, of concern regarding health care access was the difficulty being transgender created for FTMs who went for a physical, a difficulty they were more likely than MTFs to experience. A possible reason for this gender difference is that undergoing a physical may be difficult for FTMs because some female medical procedures such as pap smears, are included in the exam. Other studies have found that negative experiences in health care settings may lead people to forego seeking similar services in the future (O'Hanlan, Cabaj, Schatz, Lock, & Nemrow, 1997; O'Hanlan, 1996). For FTMs who do not identify with their female body, the idea of being treated as female can be emotionally difficult and a deterrent to obtaining a physical. Poor experiences or even negative associations with the health care system may cause FTMs, in particular, to avoid not only physicals but other necessary routine care. This could potentially contribute to heightened morbidities that are otherwise preventable or treatable. Such findings continue to highlight the need for training of health care professionals on how to provide competent care to transgender individuals (Feinberg, 2001; JSI Research & Training Institute, 2000).

The findings together demonstrate that transgender people face barriers to care, have a need for a range of service needs and have major health concerns such as HIV, suicidality, violence and barriers to service access. We caution, however, against interpreting the findings as evidence of an "illness" or "pathology" that is inherent to transgender people, such that plans of action are focused solely on "fixing" individuals. The obstacles that transgender people confront cannot be separated from the environment in which the obstacles occur. The larger social context that still sanctions discrimination and violence based upon gender identity cannot be ignored and we must acknowledge the reality of socially enforced barriers so that we can strive to dismantle them. Future efforts to meet the health and social service needs of transgender people must include macro level social change so people who challenge and seek to redefine narrowly constructed gender norms are not legally, socially, politically and medically marginalized.

REFERENCES

American Association of Suicidology (2001). U.S.A. suicide: 1999 official final data. Retrieved December 10, 2001, from *http://www.suicidology.org/index.html.*

Block, N. L., & Tessler, A. N. (1973). Transsexualism and surgical procedures. *Medical Aspects of Human Sexuality, 7,* 158-186.

Bockting, W., Beatrice, O., Robinson, B. E., & Rosser, B. R. S. (1998). Transgender HIV prevention: A qualitative needs assessment. *AIDS Care, 10,* 505-526.

Bowen, G. (1995). *Violence and health poll.* (Available from The American Boyz, P. O. Box 1118, Elkton, MD, 21922-1118).

Centers for Disease Control and Prevention. (n.d.). HIV/AIDS among US women: Minority and young women at continuing risk. Retrieved July 25, 2003, from *http://www.cdc.gov/hiv/pubs/facts/women.htm.*

Clements, K., Marx, R., Guzman, R., Ikeda, S. & Katz, M. (1998). Prevalence of HIV infection in transgendered individuals in San Francisco. Poster presented at the XII International Conference on AIDS, Geneva, Switzerland.

Clements-Nolle, K., Marx, R., Guzman, R., & Katz, M. (2001). HIV prevalence, risk behaviors, health care use, and mental health status of transgender persons: Implications for public health intervention. *American Journal of Public Health, 91,* 915-921.

Courvant, D. (1997). *Domestic violence and the sex- or gender-variant survivor.* (Available from the Survivor Project, 5028 NE 8th, Portland, OR 97211).

DiNitto, D. M. (2000). Social welfare: Politics and public policy (5th ed.). Boston: Allyn and Bacon.

Elifson, K. W., Boles, J., Posey, E., Sweat, M., Darrow, W., & Elsea, W. (1993). Male transvestite prostitutes and HIV risk. *American Journal of Public Health, 83,* 260-262.

Feinberg, L. (2001). Trans health crisis: For us it's life or death. *American Journal of Public Health, 91,* 897-900.

JSI Research & Training Institute, Inc., (2000). *Access to health care for transgendered persons in greater Boston.* Boston: GLBT Health Access Project.

Kammerer, N., Mason, T., Connors, M., & Durkee, R. (2001). Transgender health and social service needs in the context of HIV risk. In W. Bockting & S. Kirk (Eds.), *Transgender and HIV: Risks, prevention, and care* (pp. 39-57). New York: The Haworth Press, Inc.

Kammerer, N., Mason, T., Connors, M., Durkee, R. (2001). Transgender health and social service needs in the context of HIV risk. In. W. Bockting, & S. Kirk (Eds.). *Transgender and HIV: Risks, prevention, and care* (pp. 39-57). New York: The Haworth Press, Inc.

Kenagy, G. P. (2002). HIV among transgendered people. *AIDS Care, 14,* 127-134.

Kenagy, G. P. (In press). Transgender Health: Findings From Two Needs Assessment Studies in Philadelphia. *Health and Social Work.*

Levine, C. O. (1978). Social work with transsexuals. *Social Casework, 59,* 167-174.

MacKenzie, G. O. (1994). *Transgender nation.* Bowling Green, OH: Bowling Green State University Popular Press.

Namaste, V. K. (1999). HIV/AIDS and female to male transsexuals and transvestites: Results from a needs assessment in Quebec. *International Journal of Transgenderism.* Retrieved March 29, 2002, *http://www.symposion.com/itj/hiv_risk/namaste.htm.*

Namaste, K. Laframboise S., & Brady D. (n.d.). *Transgendered people and HIV/AIDS: An introduction to transgendered people's health concerns regarding HIV and AIDS.* Vancouver: High Risk Project.

National Institute of Allergy and Infectious Diseases. (December, 2002). HIV/AIDS statistics. Retrieved July 25, 2003 from, *http://www.niaid.nih.gov/factsheets/aidsstat.htm.*

O'Hanlan, K. A. (1996). Do we really mean preventive medicine for all? *American Journal of Preventive Medicine, 12,* 411-414.

O'Hanlan, K. A., Cabaj, R. J., Schatz, B., Lock, J., & Nemrow, P. (1997). A review of the medical consequences of homophobia with suggestions for resolution. *Journal of the Gay and Lesbian Medical Association, 1,* 25-39.

Reback, C. J., Simon, P. A., Bemis, C. C., & Gatson, B. (2001). *The Los Angeles transgender health study: Community report.* Los Angeles: Authors.

U.S. Department of Health and Human Services, National Center for Health Statistics. (1993). National health interview survey, 1992: AIDS knowledge and attitudes supplement [computer file]. Hyattsville, MD: U.S. Dept. of Health and Human Services, National Center for Health Statistics [producer], 1993. Ann Arbor, MI: Inter-university Consortium for Political and Social Research [distributor], 1994.

Warren, B. E. (1999). Sex, truth and videotape HIV: Prevention at the Gender Identity Project in New York City. *International Journal of Transgenderism.* Retrieved March 29, 2002, from *http://www.symposion.com/itj/hiv_risk/warren.htm.*

Wicks, L. K. (1977). Transsexualism: A social work approach. *Health and Social Work, 2,* 180-193.

Wilchins, R. A., Lombardi, E., Priesing, D., & Malouf, D. (1997). *First national survey of transgender violence.* New York: GenderPAC.

Xavier, J. M. (2000). *The Washington transgender needs assessment survey.* Retrieved January 15, 2002, from *http://www.gender.org/vaults/wtnas.html.*

Sex, Drugs, Violence, and HIV Status Among Male-to-Female Transgender Persons in Houston, Texas

Jan M. H. Risser, PhD
Andrea Shelton, PhD
Sheryl McCurdy, PhD
John Atkinson, DrPH
Paige Padgett, PhD
Bernardo Useche, PhD
Brenda Thomas
Mark Williams, PhD

SUMMARY. To inform the Community Planning Group (Houston, Texas) in setting HIV-prevention priorities, risk behavior surveys were completed by 67 male-to-female (MtF) transgender persons. By self-identification, 58% were preoperative and 48% were self-described heterosexual women. We found this small sample of male-to-female transgender individuals to have high rates of HIV infection, and high prevalence of risky behaviors, intimate partner violence, and suicidal ideation. Twenty-seven percent were infected with HIV. Barriers were seldom used during oral sex and used less than half the time for anal sex with either primary or casual partners. Nearly one-third of the sample reported use of methamphetamines, amyl nitrite or LSD and 40% reported crack or cocaine use. Intimate partner violence and forced sex were reported by 50% and 25%, respectively. Suicidal ideation was reported by 16% in the last 30 days; lifetime suicidal ideation was 60%. *[Article copies available for a fee from The Haworth Document Delivery Service: 1-800-HAWORTH. E-mail address: <docdelivery@haworthpress.com> Website: <http://www.HaworthPress.com> © 2005 by The Haworth Press, Inc. All rights reserved.]*

KEYWORDS. Transgender, HIV prevention, HIV risk, violence, drug use

Jan M. H. Risser, PhD, Andrea Shelton, PhD, Sheryl McCurdy, PhD, John Atkinson, DrPH, Paige Padgett, PhD, Bernardo Useche, PhD, and Mark Williams, PhD, are all affiliated with the School of Public Health, University of Texas Health Science Center at Houston, Houston, TX. Brenda Thomas is affiliated with the Transgender Outreach Project, Houston Department of Health and Human Services, Houston, TX.

Address correspondence to: Jan M. H. Risser, PhD, School of Public Health, University of Texas-Houston, RAS E 703, 1200 Herman Pressler, Houston, TX 77030 (E-mail: Jan.M.Risser@uth.tmc.edu).

This research was supported by a grant from The Houston Department of Health and Human Services.

The opinions expressed herein are solely those of the authors.

[Haworth co-indexing entry note]: "Sex, Drugs, Violence, and HIV Status Among Male-to-Female Transgender Persons in Houston, Texas." Risser, Jan M. H. et al. Co-published simultaneously in *International Journal of Transgenderism* (The Haworth Medical Press, an imprint of The Haworth Press, Inc.) Vol. 8, No. 2/3, 2005, pp. 67-74; and: *Transgender Health and HIV Prevention: Needs Assessment Studies from Transgender Communities Across the United States* (ed: Walter Bockting, and Eric Avery) The Haworth Medical Press, an imprint of The Haworth Press, Inc., 2005, pp. 67-74. Single or multiple copies of this article are available for a fee from The Haworth Document Delivery Service [1-800-HAWORTH, 9:00 a.m. - 5:00 p.m. (EST). E-mail address: docdelivery@haworthpress.com].

INTRODUCTION

HIV and other sexually transmitted infections are serious health concerns facing the transgender community (Bockting and Kirk, 2001). Research on this population's sexual health issues has been neglected, particularly in the United States (Boehmer, 2002).

A small study in Atlanta (Elifson et al., 1993) found that 68% of 53 transgender sex workers were HIV-positive, 81% had seromarkers for syphilis, and 80% had seromarkers for hepatitis B. Other investigators (Modan et al., 1992) conducted a qualitative study of male-to-female (MtF) transgender sex workers in Tel Aviv, Israel, and found that HIV infection rates were nearly 10 times higher (11.1%) than HIV infection rates in female commercial sex workers (1.1%). Among 22 transgender sex workers attending a drug dependency unit in Rome, 86% were HIV-positive (Gattari et al., 1991).

Clements-Nolle (Clements-Nolle et al., 2001) found a HIV prevalence of 35% among MtF transgender people. In some studies, transgender people are found to have higher risk of HIV/AIDS than men who have sex with men (MSM). The prevalence of HIV among African American MtF transgender people may be as high as 60% (Lombardi, 2001) and the incidence has been reported to be 7.8 new cases per 100 person years of follow-up (Kellogg et al., 2001).

Little is known about behavioral risks of MtF transgender persons in Houston, Texas, including the size of the population. We have estimated that the transgender population in Houston is between 1,000 to 16,000 individuals based on prevalence data from other studies. Prevalence of MtF transgender persons is reported to be 5.5 per 100,000 to 32.5 per 100,000 when describing the proportion seeking hormonal therapy, sex-reassignment surgery, or psychiatric support (Eklund et al., 1988, Tsoi, 1988, van Kesteren et al., 1996, Bakker et al., 1993, Weitze and Osburg, 1996, Wilson et al., 1999). This research was designed to describe behavioral risks of MtF transgender individuals in Houston, TX, in an effort to inform priority-setting functions of the HIV Prevention Community Planning Group.

METHODS

Sample

Participants were recruited through a network of transgender service organizations, and through bars and clubs identified by key informants. Recruitment was by study personnel or referral by transgender individuals who had already participated in the project. Of the 67 MtF transgender individuals interviewed, 23 were recruited from bars, 15 from transgender support groups, and 29 by referrals. Data collection took place during December 2002 and January 2003.

The UT/SPH Institutional Review Board reviewed procedures and data collection instruments and granted permission to conduct the study. Participants were verbally informed of the objectives of the study.

Instrument

The questions for the survey instrument were developed in September of 2002 with the collaboration of researchers conducting similar rapid needs assessments with other high-risk populations in Houston (HDHHS, 2003). The questionnaire was then refined by the investigators at the University of Texas School of Public Health (UT/SPH) who were working with the transgender population.

The survey included: basic demographic information, sexual identity and orientation, HIV risk behaviors related to sexual behavior and drug use, the social context of these behaviors, history of sexually transmitted infections (STIs) and HIV testing, HIV status, issues related to forced sex, domestic violence, and history of suicidal thoughts and attempts.

Procedure

Three interviewers were trained to administer the survey by two methods. In the field office, computer assisted personal interviews (CAPI) were conducted using Questionnaire Design Studio (QDS) software (NOVA Research Company, Bethesda, Maryland); paper interviews were used at the other recruitment venues. The interviews took about 20-30 minutes to complete. In order to provide more nuanced detail about individual lives and experiences, the interviewers recorded comments and field notes. Agreeing to participate in the interview was considered consent. Individuals were offered a small monetary incentive for participating and additional incentive for recruiting other respondents.

Data Analysis

Data management and statistical analysis were conducted with SPSS 11.0.1. Basic descriptive statistics were utilized and statistical significance was assessed using Chi-square tests where appropriate.

RESULTS

Characteristics of the Sample

Characteristics of the sample are presented in Table 1. One-half described themselves as heterosexual women (MtF transgender with male sexual partners) and another 11% described themselves as lesbian (MtF transgender with female sexual partners). Age ranged from 18 to 45 years; the median age was 35 years, and 69% were under age 40. The sample was 46% Anglo, 30% African American, and 20% Hispanic; this approximates the Houston/Harris County 2003 population which is 40% Anglo, 18% African American, and 35% Hispanic. While one-fifth of the sample had not graduated from high school, two-fifths had attended or graduated from college. Approximately one-half were employed full or part-time.

Field Notes–Unique Characteristics

In addition to the results shown in Table 1, it is relevant to emphasize the wide scope of sexual orientation categories found in this study. One individual defined herself as asexual because she is attracted to no one. Some self-identified as bisexuals, others as heterosexual males, heterosexual females, homosexual males, and homosexual females. In addition, many expressed that they felt very confused and concerned about how to categorize their sexual orientation.

For some individuals, describing personal gender identity and sexual orientation can be complex. For example, a Drag Queen considered himself a homosexual male who cross-dresses for fun. Another interviewee, a post-operative MtF prostitute, self-identified as a homosexual male who underwent sex reassignment surgery only because he wanted to have access to a higher number of male heterosexual clients.

Sexually Transmitted Infections and HIV

Twenty-eight (42%) participants reported a previous diagnosis of syphilis, gonorrhea, genital warts, genital herpes, or chlamydia (Table 2). For gonorrhea, syphilis, and herpes, more than 70% of cases were treated in public rather than private clinics. Among those treated for syphilis and/or gonorrhea, when asked: "Do you consider yourself cured" of your infection,

TABLE 1. Sample Characteristics

	n	%
Race/Ethnicity (N = 67)		
African American	20	30%
Anglo/White	31	46%
Hispanic/Latino	13	19%
Other	3	5%
Education (N = 67)		
Less than high school	14	21%
High school diploma or vocational training	24	36%
Some college or college degree	29	43%
Employment (N = 67)		
Employed	31	46%
Unemployed	27	40%
Disabled	6	9%
Other	3	5%
Self-Reported Gender Identity (N = 67)		
Male	4	6%
Female	17	25%
Male-to-Female preoperative	39	58%
Male-to-Female postoperative	7	10%
Sexual Orientation (N = 66)		
Heterosexual	32	48%
Bisexual	17	26%
Homosexual male (gay)	10	15%
Homosexual female (lesbian)	7	11%

TABLE 2. History of Sexually Transmitted Infections

	n	%
Sexually Transmitted Infection (N = 67)		
Gonorrhea	7	10%
Syphilis	14	21%
Genital herpes	4	6%
Chlamydia	3	4%
Genital warts	7	10%
Any STD	28	42%
Do not feel cured of disease	6	9%

10% reported that they did not feel cured, even though they reported that they had completed treatment.

Sixty-two participants (93%) had been tested for HIV (Table 3), including 67% in the last year. Fifty-two of these 62 individuals (84%) had received the results of their last HIV test. One participant reported results that were indeterminate. Of the remaining 51, 14 (27%) were HIV positive. Each of the five who had never been tested believed they were HIV negative. Reasons for not getting tested included: a belief that one was negative, a feeling that one did not engage in risky behavior, and the fact that one had only one partner. We did not collect information on why individuals did not seek test results.

Alcohol and Drug Use

Almost all MtFs in the sample had used alcohol and nearly three-quarters reported marijuana use at some time in their lives (Table 4). More than 40% reported crack cocaine or powder cocaine use, and nearly one-third reported use of one or more of the following: LSD, methamphetamines, and poppers (amyl nitrite). Twenty percent reported previous use of Ecstasy (3,4-Methylenedioxymethamphetamine). Ten percent or less reported previous use of heroin, Viagra (Sildenafil), Special K (ketamine), and/or GHB (gamma hydroxybutyrate).

Fifty participants (75%) had used feminizing hormones at some point in their lives; the majority started before age 26 years. Thirty-seven (55%) had used hormones at least once in the previous 30 days (median use = 30.0 times, mean = 25.2, SD = 18.1). Among the 30-day us-

ers, 65% reported they had injected hormones at some time in their lives.

Twenty-seven persons (40%) reported injection drug use in their lifetime; of these, twelve (44%) had injected within the last month. The number of times injected in the last 30 days ranged from 1 to 200 (median = 5.0, mean = 25.2, SD = 55.7). Four of those interviewed, or 33% of 30-day injectors had shared needles, cookers, cotton, and/or water.

Nine participants (13%) had ever received a silicone injection. Of these, three (33%) stated that they never used sterile needles for these injections.

Sexual Behavior

Primary Partner

Twenty-six participants (39%) reported having a current primary partner (Table 5). Primary partner was defined as "one considered to be like a husband, wife, or lover." Of those with a primary partner, 69% reported that their primary partner was male. One-half had oral sex with their primary partner at least once in the last thirty days, 12 (45%) had anal sex, and four (15%) had vaginal sex. Most participants (69%) reported never using barriers during oral sex with their current primary partner; and only 50% reported always using male condoms during anal sex. However, 58% of those who had anal sex reported using a male condom the last time they had anal sex. Eighteen (69%) of those participants with a current primary partner reported using alcohol or drugs at their last sexual encounter.

Casual Partner

Thirty-three MtF transgender individuals (49%) reported having at least one casual partner dur-

TABLE 3. HIV Testing

	n	%
Ever had HIV test (N = 67)	62	93%
Acquired Results	52	84%
HIV test results (N = 52)		
Positive	14	27%
Negative	37	71%
Indeterminate	1	2%

TABLE 4. Alcohol and Drug Use

N = 67	Ever Used		Used in Last 30 Days		Used in Last 7 Days	
	n	%	n	%	n	%
Alcohol	65	97%	51	76%	46	69%
Marijuana	49	73%	20	30%	16	24%
Crack Cocaine	30	45%	22	33%	20	30%
Powder Cocaine	30	45%	9	13%	6	9%
LSD/Acid	22	33%	0	0%	0	0%
Poppers/Rush (alkyl nitrate)	21	31%	2	3%	1	2%
Methamphetamines	19	28%	3	4%	1	2%
Ecstasy/X/E	13	19%	3	4%	2	3%
Heroin	7	10%	2	3%	1	2%
Viagra	6	9%	3	4%	1	2%
Special K	5	7%	0	0%	0	0%
GHB	2	3%	0	0%	0	0%
Hormones	50	75%	37	55%	32	48%
Silicone*	9	13%				

*Information on 30 day and 7 day silicone use was not collected.

TABLE 5. Self-Reported Sexual Behavior with Primary Partners

	n	%
Had primary partner in last 12 months (N = 67)	47	70%
Currently have a primary partner (N = 67)	26	39%
Gender identity of primary partner (N = 26)		
Male	18	69%
Female	6	23%
Transgender	2	8%
Alcohol or drug use during sex with primary partner (N = 23)		
Never	52	22%
Sometimes	46	70%
Always	2	9%
Had a casual partner in past 12 months (N = 67)	33	49%
Had a casual partner in last 30 days (N = 66)	25	38%

ing the last year and 25 (37%) during the last 30 days (Table 5). Of those reporting a casual partner in the last 30 days, 92% reported that partner to be male, 4% reported female casual partners, and 24% reported transgender casual partners (sum is greater than 100% because in-

dividuals may report both male and female or transgender partners). Sexual behavior with a casual partner in the last 30 days was reported as: 84% engaging in oral sex; 84% anal sex; and 4% vaginal sex. Barriers were never used by 43% of those reporting oral sex and 33% of those reporting anal sex.

Field Notes–Sexual Behaviors

The sample included transgender persons who had been celibate for more than one year, others who had continued in a sexually monogamous relationship with their wives after transition to a female role, and those who worked in prostitution and might have had sex with as many as 40 or 50 different partners a week. Two categories of the latter were evident: there was a clear differentiation between the majority, who were street workers and seemed to have little power for negotiating protective behaviors, and a minority who ran their own websites, advertised themselves in local newspapers, or owned business such as massage services. The latter group reported that they had the opportunity to screen clients and to exercise control over condom use.

One-half of participants had traded sex for money, and one-fifth had traded money for sex. One-quarter reported trading sex for drugs, and 12% had traded drugs for sex (Table 6).

While the ability to assess the significance of the relationships between participants' HIV risk behaviors and HIV status is limited by the sample size, some significant relationships were noted. For example, 40% of those who had ever used crack were HIV positive compared to 15% of those who had not ($\chi_1^2 = 3.88$, p = 0.05). Sixty-two percent (62%) of those who had ever traded sex for drugs were HIV positive compared to 15% of those who had not ($\chi_1^2 = 10.3$, p = 0.001). Eighty percent of those who had ever traded drugs for sex reported they were in-

TABLE 6. Self-Reported Exchange of Sex or Drugs for Money

	n	%
Ever traded sex for money (N = 67)	34	51%
Ever traded money for sex (N = 67)	13	19%
Ever traded sex for drugs (N = 62)	16	26%
Ever traded drugs for sex (N = 61)	7	12%

fected compared to 22% who had not engaged is such a trade ($\chi_1^2 = 7.4$, p = 0 .006).

Partner Violence and Suicidal Ideation

Lifetime prevalence of partner violence and self-inflicted harm was ascertained. Twenty-five percent reported forced sex, and 50% had been hit by a primary partner. Sixteen percent reported forced sex, and 22% had been hit by a casual sex partner. Nearly 60% had thought about suicide at some point in their lives. Eleven of those interviewed (16%) had thought about suicide in the last 30 days. Thirty percent (20/67) reported at least one suicide attempt.

DISCUSSION

The reported prevalence of HIV infection in our sample confirms the high rate of HIV found by other U.S. and international studies of transgender sex workers who have found rates of HIV to range from 11% to 86% (Elifson et al., 1993, Modan et al., 1992, Gattari et al., 1991). Since this was a sample of convenience, it would be inappropriate to generalize the findings from this study to the entire transgender population of Houston. However, our findings do seem to support a high burden of HIV infection, and high risk of infection in segments of the Houston transgender community.

The high HIV prevalence found is congruent with the risk behaviors of the interviewees who reported unprotected sexual activity, drug use, and survival sex, as found in other studies with transgender populations (Clements et al., 1999). The rate of unprotected anal sex reported in this study (50%) for MtF transgender persons is similar to that found among MSM (Koblin et al., 2003) where 48% reported unprotected receptive anal sex, and 55% unprotected insertive anal sex. HIV prevalence was also significantly associated with having used crack and having traded sex for drugs or drugs for sex.

Reported motivation for MSMs who are infected with HIV to use methamphetamines, alcohol, and other drugs during sex is the effect these substances have in making it easier to find anonymous partners, enhancing sexual pleasure, and coping with situations related to their HIV status (Semple et al., 2002). This is a reasonable explanation for the rates of drug use reported by MtF transgender individuals in our survey.

Drug use has also been noted in association with violence. Higher rates of drug use, namely alcohol and marijuana, were reported among MtF transgender sex workers in association with physical assault compared to female counterparts in studies conducted in Hawaii and Washington, D.C. (Valera et al., 2001, Odo and Hawelu, 2001).

Reported cases of violence were high in our study. The prevalence of intimate partner abuse in lesbian, gay, bisexual and transgender communities ranges between 25%-40%, comparable to national rates for heterosexual couples (Harms, 1995, Lockhart et al., 1994, Koss et al., 1987, Brand and Kidd, 1986). Nationally, higher rates of domestic violence have been documented among MtF transgender persons compared to non-transgender females (National Coalition of Anti-Violence Programs, 2000). The range of reported battery by an intimate partner in studies of transgender individuals is 20%-50% (Cook-Daniels, 1997, Odo and Hawelu, 2001). Results of our present study suggest a higher prevalence of victimization by a primary partner in comparison to national findings for heterosexuals and the LGBT communities collectively, but one consistent with the range suggested in other studies of transgender people.

Suicide attempts and completed suicides are commonly reported among transgender people, and rates for both are higher than the general population (Semple et al., 2002, van Kesteren et al., 1996, Dean et al., 2000). Rates in the present study exceed those in other samples of transgender individuals, however (Xavier, 2000, Clements-Nolle et al., 2001, Pfafflin and Junge, 1992, Dixon et al., 1984). Suicide rates are noted to decline among transgender persons after sex reassignment surgery (Dean et al., 2000). An analysis of self-inflicted violence after surgery is beyond the scope of this study because so few had undergone the procedure.

Thirteen percent of our sample reported to have had silicone injections from people who did not have medical licenses. Our field notes show that the main motivation for such practice is the low comparative cost with respect to cosmetic surgery and the immediate feminizing effect. Silicone injections administered by unlicensed practitioners can cause serious health complications. In Houston during the summer of 2003, three transgender individuals died from such illegal injections (O'hare, 2003). Educating the transgender community about the dangers of industrial grade silicone injections by unlicensed personnel could save lives.

From our field notes and observations, we identified several needs among the study participants. One need was related to the transition process common to the transgender population: few received appropriate attention to their transition issues as prescribed by the Standards of Care for Gender Disorders (Meyer III et al., 2001). Some felt angry about a society that discriminates against them, whereas others felt depressed because they could not afford the hormones, medical procedures, or surgeries that their condition requires. After having been off hormones for six months, one of the respondents complained that hair was starting to grow again on her chest, that the size of her breasts had decreased, and that her penis "has come back to life." In addition, she reported that her voice had become deeper, which she attributed to having been off her hormones, even though feminizing hormones do not have a known effect on the voice. In this context, initiatives oriented to offer social support as well as medical, psychological and other services could be instrumental in the implementation of health care programs that benefit the transgender community.

Other needs identified were directly related to HIV/STDs prevention issues. The street workers asked for condoms. One of them disclosed that she had been recently diagnosed with syphilis and had not received effective treatment. She was eager to be referred to a doctor or clinic and to receive education about STD prevention. Another, who several weeks ago had tested HIV-negative, said: "until now I've been lucky, but I know that being a whore I am going to die of AIDS."

CONCLUSION

In the same way that the term MSM is used in order to avoid categorizing male homosexuality as a risk factor for HIV/AIDS, it is extremely important to avoid the labeling of any transgender identity or sexual orientation as a risk factor for HIV transmission. Using the appropriate terms to identify the particular behaviors, attitudes and situations that put transgender people and their social networks at risk, we can develop interventions to reduce HIV transmission in this population.

Future studies should assess the links between HIV risk behaviors, including drug use and domestic violence. In addition, future studies in Houston need to identify the HIV and STI prevention messages that would be most appropriate for the transgender community.

REFERENCES

Bakker, A., van Kesteren, P., Gooren, L. and Bezemer, P. (1993) The prevalence of transsexualism in the Netherlands. *Acta Psychiatrica Scandinavica, 87,* 237-238.

Bockting, W. O. and Kirk, S. (2001) *Transgender and HIV: Risks, prevention, and care,* The Haworth Press, Inc.: Binghamton, NY.

Boehmer, U. (2002) Twenty years of public health research: Inclusion of lesbian, gay, bisexual, and transgender populations. *American Journal of Public Health, 92,* 1125-30.

Brand, P. and Kidd, A. (1986) Frequency of physical aggression in heterosexual and female homosexual dyads. *Psychological Reports, 59,* 1307-1313.

Clements, K., Wilkinson, W., Kitano, K. and Marx, R. (1999) HIV Prevention and Health Service Needs of the Transgender Community in San Francisco. *http://www.symposion.com/ijt/hiv_risk/clements.htm.*

Clements-Nolle, K., Marx, R., Guzman, R. and Katz, M. (2001) HIV prevalence, risk behaviors, health care use, and mental health status of transgender persons: Implications for public health intervention. *American Journal of Public Health, 91,* 915-21.

Cook-Daniels, L. (1997) Lesbian, Gay Male, Bisexual and Transgendered Elders: Elder Abuse and Neglect Issues. *Journal of Elder Abuse & Neglect, 9,* 35-49.

Dean, L., Meyer, I., Robinson, K., Sell, R., Sember, R., Silenzio, V., Bowen, D., Bradford, J., Rothblum, E., Scout, M. A., White, J., Dunn, P., Lawrence, A., Wolfe, D. and Xavier, J. (2000) Lesbian, gay, bisexual, and transgender health: Findings and concerns.

Journal of the Gay and Lesbian Medical Association, 4, 101-151.

Dixon, J., Maddever, H. and Van Maasden, J. (1984) Psychosocial characteristics of applicants evaluated for surgical gender reassignment. *Archives of Sexual Behavior, 13,* 269-277.

Eklund, P., Gooren, L. and Bezemer, P. (1988) Prevalence of transsexualism in the Netherlands. *British Journal of Psychiatry, 152,* 638-40.

Elifson, K. W., Boles, J., Posey, E., Sweat, M., Darrow, W. and Elsea, W. (1993) Male transvestite prostitutes and HIV risk. *American Journal of Public Health, 83,* 260-2.

Gattari, P., Rezza, G., Zaccarelli, M., Valenzi, C. and Tirelli, U. (1991) HIV infection in drug using transvestites and transsexuals. [letter to the editor]. *European Journal of Epidemiology, 7,* 711-712.

Harms, B. (1995) Domestic violence in the gay male community. *Unpublished Master's thesis. San Francisco State University, Department of Psychology.*

HDHHS (2003) Houston Department of Health and Human Services Bureau of HIV/STD Prevention. Reports on Behavioral Rapid Need Assessments of ten populations at risk for HIV/STD infections. Unpublished report to the Community Planning Group, Houston, Texas.

Kellogg, T. A., Clements-Nolle, K., Dilley, J., Katz, M. H. and McFarland, W. (2001) Incidence of human immunodeficiency virus among male-to-female transgendered persons in San Francisco. *Journal of Acquired Immune Deficiency Syndromes, 28,* 380-4.

Koblin, B., Chesney, M., Husnik, M., Bozeman, S., Celum, C., Buchbinder, S., Mayer, K., McKirnan, D., Judson, F., Huang, Y. and Coates, T. (2003) High-risk behaviors among men who have sex with men in 6 US cities: Baseline data from the EXPLORE Study. *American Journal of Public Health, 93,* 926-932.

Koss, M., Gidycz, C. and Wisneiswki, N. (1987) The scope of rape: Incidence and prevalence of sexual aggression and victimization in a national sample of higher education students. *Journal of Consulting Clinical Psychology, 55,* 162-170.

Lockhart, L., White, B., Causby, V. and Tsaac, A. (1994) Letting out the secret: Violence in lesbian relationships. *The Journal of Interpersonal Violence, 9,* 469-492.

Lombardi, E. (2001) Enhancing transgender health care. *American Journal of Public Health, 91,* 869-72.

Meyer III, W., Bockting, W., Cohen-Kettenis, P., Coleman, E., DiCeglie, D., Devor, H., Gooren, L., Joris Hage, J., Kirk, S., Kuiper, B., Laub, D., Lawrence, A., Menard, Y., Patton, J., Schaefer, L., Webb, A. and Wheeler, C. (2001) The Standards of Care for Gender Identity Disorders–Sixth Version. *International Journal of Transgenderism, 5,* http://www.symposion.com/ijt/soc_2001/index.htm.

Modan, B., Goldschmidt, R., Rubinstein, E., Vonsover, A., Zinn, M., Golan, R., Chetrit, A. and Gottlieb-Stematzky, T. (1992) Prevalence of HIV antibodies in transsexual and female prostitutes. *American Journal of Public Health, 82,* 590-2.

National Coalition of Anti-Violence Programs (2000) Lesbian, Gay, Bisexual, and Transgender Domestic Violence in 2000. Preliminary Edition.

Odo, C. and Hawelu, A. (2001) Eo na Mahu of Hawai'i: The extraordinary health needs of Hawai'i's Mahu. *Pacific Health Dialog, 8,* 327-334.

O'hare, P. (2003) In *Houston Chronicle,* Houston, Texas.

Pfafflin, F. and Junge, A. (1992) *Sex Reassignment: Thirty Years of International Follow-up Studies After SRS–A Comprehensive Review, 1961-1991, Schattau*er: Stuttgart.

Semple, S., Patterson, T. and Grant, I. (2002) Motivations associated with methamphetamine use among HIV+ men who have sex with men. *Journal of Substance Abuse Treatment, 22,* 149-156.

Tsoi, W. (1988) The prevalence of transsexualism in Singapore. *Acta Psychiatrica Scandinavica, 78,* 501-4.

Valera, R. J., Sawyer, R. G. and Schiraldi, G. R. (2001) Perceived health needs of inner-city street prostitutes: A preliminary study. *American Journal of Health Behavior, 25,* 50-9.

van Kesteren, P., Gooren, J. and Megens, J. (1996) An epidemiological and demographic study of transsexuals in the Netherlands. *Archives of Sexual Behavior, 25,* 589-600.

Weitze, C. and Osburg, S. (1996) Transsexualism in Germany: empirical data on epidemiology and application of the German Transsexuals' Act during its first ten years. *Archives of Sexual Behavior, 25,* 409-25.

Wilson, P., Sharp, C. and Carr, S. (1999) The prevalence of gender dysphoria in Scotland: A primary care study. *British Journal of General Practice, 49,* 991-992.

Xavier, J. M. (2000) HIV and AIDS Administration, Government of the District of Columbia.

Access to Health Care for Transgendered Persons: Results of a Needs Assessment in Boston

Jodi Sperber, MSW, MPH
Stewart Landers, JD, MCP
Susan Lawrence, MA

SUMMARY. The transgender community is a population group that has experienced an increase in visibility, with only a small, concomitant increase in understanding. This study reports on four focus groups, in which 34 transgendered individuals discussed their experiences and interactions with the health care system.

The specific aims of the study were as follows:

- Identify the health needs of transgender and transsexual (TG/TS) individuals;
- Hear the experiences and perceptions of TG/TS individuals who are using the current health care system;
- Identify any barriers to obtaining services, support and/or resources;
- Assess the extent to which health care providers and systems are able to offer sensitive, high quality and user friendly services that meet TG/TS consumers' needs; and
- Identify ways that health care services can be enhanced to better meet the needs of the target population.

What the study found was a system that was anything but high quality in meeting the needs of TG/TS individuals. Ignorance, insensitivity and discrimination appear to be the norm. Specifically, the focus groups found the following:

- Transgendered and transsexual persons frequently encounter providers who will not treat them and blatantly say so. There is a need for education and a change in anti-discrimination law needed to change this.
- The lack of provider training on transgender issues creates insensitivity to simple issues of respect for trans people. One example is the unwillingness to address TG/TS people by the pronoun preferred by the patient/client.

Jodi Sperber, MSW, MPH, was affiliated with John Snow, Inc. when this article was written. She is now affiliated with Health Dialog, Manchester, NH. Stewart Landers, JD, MCP, and Susan Lawrence, MA, are both affiliated with John Snow, Inc., JSI Research and Training Institute, Inc., Boston, MA.

The authors would like to thank all of the transgender and transsexual individuals who participated in these focus groups. Special thanks to the group facilitators: Rebecca Durkee, Dean Kotula, Alejandro Marcel, Jessica Piper and Grace Stowell. Michele Clark trained the facilitators. Gary Fallas and Jodi Sperber assisted with the organizing of the focus groups and served as note takers.

[Haworth co-indexing entry note]: "Access to Health Care for Transgendered Persons: Results of a Needs Assessment in Boston." Sperber, Jodi, Stewart Landers, and Susan Lawrence. Co-published simultaneously in *International Journal of Transgenderism* (The Haworth Medical Press, an imprint of The Haworth Press, Inc.) Vol. 8, No. 2/3, 2005, pp. 75-91; and: *Transgender Health and HIV Prevention: Needs Assessment Studies from Transgender Communities Across the United States* (ed: Walter Bockting, and Eric Avery) The Haworth Medical Press, an imprint of The Haworth Press, Inc., 2005, pp. 75-91. Single or multiple copies of this article are available for a fee from The Haworth Document Delivery Service [1-800-HAWORTH, 9:00 a.m. - 5:00 p.m. (EST). E-mail address: docdelivery@haworthpress.com].

Available online at http://www.haworthpress.com/web/IJT
doi:10.1300/J485v08n02_08

- Many providers lack the knowledge to adequately treat many of the routine health care needs of TG/TS individuals when such treatment relates to issues of hormone use, gynecological care, HIV prevention counseling, or other concerns related to gender or sexuality.
- Providers frequently refer to trans issues in unrelated health care situations such as setting a broken bone, filling a cavity or treating a cold. Greater familiarity with the health care needs of the trans population would reduce such incidents.
- Mental health and substance abuse treatment providers need additional training in order to work cooperatively with TG/TS clients to identify when gender issues are or are not relevant to specific mental health or substance abuse treatment episodes. Sometimes gender issues are central to mental health or substance abuse treatment, sometimes they are peripheral and sometimes they are unrelated.
- Discrimination in health insurance is the rule, not the exception. There is a need for education to encourage policy changes on the part of insurers and public policy changes on the part of legislators and regulators. *[Article copies available for a fee from The Haworth Document Delivery Service: 1-800-HAWORTH. E-mail address: <docdelivery@haworthpress.com> Website: <http://www.HaworthPress.com> © 2005 by The Haworth Press, Inc. All rights reserved.]*

KEYWORDS. Transgender, needs assessmnet, TG/TS, health care

INTRODUCTION

In recent years, gender identity issues and transgender and transsexual (TG/TS, or trans) people have received unprecedented attention in research literature as well as in the popular media. Because trans individuals may experience gender discrimination along with discrimination based on sexual orientation, they in many ways fit under the larger umbrella of a gay, lesbian, bisexual, and transgender (GLBT) community. However, in the past five years, some research has focused specifically on the unique concerns and needs of TG/TS individuals ("Health Concerns . . . ,"1997; Clements, Wilkinson et al., 1999; Clements 1999; Mason et al., 1995). It is clear from these most recent investigations that individuals who identify as trans face discrimination and other barriers, particularly in accessing health services.

Recent estimates vary as to the prevalence of transsexuality in the general population. In the United States, prevalence is estimated by the American Psychiatric Association's Diagnostic and Statistical Manual IV (1987) at 1/30,000 (born) males and 1/100,000 (born) females. In the Netherlands (1993), 1/11,900 (born) males and 1/30,400 (born) females were estimated as transsexual (Bakker et al., 1993). The discrepancy between U.S. and Dutch estimates may be related to the greater availability of care for transsexual health needs in the Netherlands and/or the greater likelihood of transgendered individuals reporting their condition there.

What gaps in health care exist for TG/TS individuals, and how can they be filled? What can providers and agencies do to make a TG/TS individual feel welcome and BE well cared for? What resources are available to providers, agencies, and consumers to facilitate high quality health care for trans people? To explore these questions, the Gay, Lesbian, Bisexual and Transgender Health Access Project (GLBT HAP) commissioned JSI Research and Training Institute, Inc. (JSI), a research and consulting firm based in Boston, Massachusetts, to conduct focus groups addressing the health care experiences and needs of TG/TS individuals. The GLBT HAP is a collaborative, community-based program funded by the Massachusetts Department of Public Health (MDPH). The program's mission is to foster the development and implementation of comprehensive, culturally appropriate, high quality health promotion policies and health care services for gay, lesbian, bisexual and transgender people and their families.

A review of current literature reveals a growing body of knowledge regarding the concerns and needs of the TG/TS community. Most of the relevant research examines HIV prevention and services, commonly by studying male-to-female (MTF) transgender or transsexual individuals (Clements, Wilkinson et al., 1999;

Clements, 1999; Mason et al., 1995). The research shows that trans individuals are at high risk for acquiring HIV. MTF individuals appear to be at particularly high risk; in one study, 35% of MTF study participants tested positive for HIV, compared to 1.6% of female-to-male (FTM) participants. Additionally, within the MTF population surveyed, African-Americans were disproportionately affected, with 63% testing positive for HIV (Clements, 1999).

While the existing research helps to identify the trans population as a group at risk for HIV infection, it also suggests that TG/TS people may be a generally ill-served or underserved population in terms of health care. Questions that arise from previous research, include "What factors contribute to the high reported HIV infection rate among trans people?" and "Do the HIV infection rates suggest that trans individuals are at a higher risk for other types of physical, emotional, or material suffering?" The high rate of HIV infection may be an indicator of broader difficulties that trans people face in accessing health care.

This study aimed to improve the health care received by trans people by exploring what a TG/TS person experiences when she or he seeks health care. The study asked participants in four focus groups to report on their experiences in obtaining routine health care as well as specialty services, and to discuss their health insurance status.

The specific aims of the study were as follows:

- Identify the health needs of transgender and transsexual (TG/TS) individuals;
- Hear the experiences and perceptions of TG/TS individuals who are using the current health care system;
- Identify any barriers to obtaining services, support and/or resources;
- Assess the extent to which health care providers and systems are able to offer sensitive, high quality and user friendly services that meet TG/TS consumers' needs; and
- Identify ways that health care services can be enhanced to better meet the needs of the target population.

METHODS

Participants were recruited for four focus groups using networking within the transgender and transsexual (TG/TS) community and outreach to health care providers who have trans clients. Advertising in community centers and health centers and outreach on the Internet drew additional participants. JSI Research and Training Institute, Inc. (JSI) managed the logistics for the focus groups, including training TG/TS community members to be the group facilitators.

Decision to Hold Four Groups

Having identified the trans community as an underserved group, the study explored how to organize focus groups to adequately represent the trans community. Networking among TG/TS people and organizations revealed the difficulty of establishing a singular trans community. The TG/TS world lacks a standard set of definitions, as the language for describing nuances of trans identity is dynamic, not fixed. The task of categorizing individual TG/TS people proved challenging, as potential study participants varied widely in terms of how they categorize themselves.

Two transgendered people who are activists for TG/TS issues in Boston aided in determining a meaningful and achievable structure for this study. These two individuals recommended that separate focus groups be conducted for MTF and FTM trans individuals. They also suggested grouping participants by age, since the perspectives and experience of youth and adults were likely to differ significantly due to the vastly greater resources available now to trans youth and the cultural/political changes as well as medical advances that have occurred over time. For example, the study anticipated age-related differences in participants' experience with hormone use and sex reassignment surgery (SRS).

It was agreed that the most important variable around which to build focus groups should be TG/TS identity. However, trans identity by its very nature belongs to an individual for whom traditional gender definitions may not fit. "Transgender" is often used as an umbrella term, and encompasses a range of identities. Individuals who choose to undergo medical procedures to alter their bodies often refer to themselves as transsexual, but this is not universally true. Because of the finite allowable number of focus groups, the gender identity categories in this study were limited to two key groups: MTF and FTM. It was acknowledged that this strategy would tend to exclude biologically inter-sexed and/or self-identified ungendered individuals. Another consideration was that people who identify as trans*sexual* might see themselves as strictly male or female, and thus different from those who identify in a less polarized fashion. Nevertheless, each focus group was likely to comprise two sub-cohorts (trans-sexual and transgender).

Some transgender and transsexual individuals (regardless of surgical status) now see themselves only in their new or current gender identity. For example, an MTF might just identify as "female" rather than "trans." Despite the possibility of discomfort between members of these two sub-cohorts, merging both groups allowed the study to examine what were potentially very different health care needs and experiences (see "Results," below). Four focus groups were planned, each determined by trans identity and age, as follows:

- Adult male-to-female (MTF);
- Adult female-to-male (FTM);
- Youth male-to-female (MTF); and
- Youth female-to-male (FTM).

A youth was defined as someone age 25 or under.

Selection of Facilitators and Participants

The groups were structured to be facilitated by trans individuals from the local community in order to build trust among focus group participants and to ensure the integrity of the study. Facilitators were sought who had experience in leading groups. Ideally, the study would have engaged only facilitators with prior experience leading groups; however, this was not feasible; therefore community leaders were carefully selected and trained in facilitation skills to help lead these groups. JSI staff experienced in training and technical assistance in focus group methodology led this training, and remained

available for questions or concerns throughout the duration of the project. A facilitator was chosen for each group who had the same MTF or FTM self-designation as that group' participants. All of the selected facilitators were adults.

Facilitators were asked to recruit community members to participate in the focus groups. Facilitators were encouraged to be open to group participants whose self-identity differed from theirs; for example, a transsexual facilitator needed to be open to people who identify as transgender. For both of the adult groups (MTF and FTM), the facilitators were able to recruit all the participants. For the MTF youth, the adult facilitator had experience working with GLBT youth and personally knew many potential participants, but would have been unable on her own to recruit a group of the size and diversity that eventually participated. A transgender female with many youth contacts helped to recruit participants. JSI staff recruited most of the participants for the FTM youth group. The facilitator was a transgender adult who works with TG/TS youth and is the director of a local transgender agency. A JSI staff person served as a note taker at each group.

A focus group moderator's guide was developed with assistance from the facilitators. This guide elicited a conversation about what participants viewed as good health care, past and present relationships with health care providers, specific services being accessed, and how a trans identity may or may not impact health-seeking behaviors.

Training of Facilitators

JSI staff trained the facilitators on qualitative research, interviewing and listening skills, preparing for and conducting a focus group, managing problematic group members and improving interviewing techniques. Elements of the training, along with feedback from the trainees, were later incorporated into a focus group facilitation guide tailored to this study.

Even with appropriate training for community-based facilitators, some bias was risked by intentionally assigning community members to help form and lead focus groups on issues crucial to their own lives. Also, while using community members to recruit and facilitate was expected to increase the comfort level and openness of a focus group, in some ways such a strategy might backfire. It was possible that focus group participants might be reluctant to share personal stories or perspectives if fellow participants belonged to the same community and might be encountered again in a different context.

RESULTS

Results summarize the aggregated findings from all four groups and are organized according to the topics discussed in each group, although not all groups discussed all of the topics below, nor did every group necessarily discuss these topics in the same order. The topics included the following:

- Identity and demographic information;
- Disclosure of TG/TS identity;
- Health issues;
- Quality and standards of care;
- Accessing health care;
- Relationships with health care providers; and
- Participant recommendations.

Identity and Demographic Information

MTF Adults

In the MTF adult group, most of the 14 participants lived in Boston. Most of the participants were white; one was Asian and one was multi-racial. Mean age was 37.

Half of the participants identified themselves as transgender and the other half chose the term transsexual. In terms of sexual orientation, 11 participants identified as heterosexual, two said they were gay, and one said she was lesbian. One identified as post-operative.

FTM Adults

The FTM adult group had 12 participants with an average age of 36. All participants completed screening instruments at the group meeting. Eleven were white and one was Latino. Nine lived in the Metro Boston area. Most of the FTM adults–regardless of their interest in or experience with sex reassignment surgery or

hormone treatment–described their sex or gender identity as transsexual (as opposed to transgender).

Five of the participants identified their sexual orientation as heterosexual, four as bisexual, and three as gay (one specifying both gay and queer). All participants in the FTM adult group said they had health insurance and a primary care doctor. Nine of the 12 said they had undergone procedures "that would be considered to be part of sex reassignment or gender reassignment."

MTF Youth

The MTF youth group included nine participants between the ages of 16 and 26 with an average age of 21. Three identified themselves as black; two as white; one as Asian (Korean); and three as other (one "biracial black and white," one "Middle Eastern/African-American," and one "Italian and Jamaican"). Five said they were employed, three said they were students, and one did not name an occupation. Eight lived in Boston.

Six participants described their sexual orientation as heterosexual, and three described theirs as gay, queer or other. Among the MTF youth, four said they were "currently taking hormones prescribed by a professional health care provider." Of the other five, two said they receive hormones from other sources, three said they did not take hormones at all, and one did not respond. Four said they had had "a procedure that would be considered to be part of sex reassignment or gender reassignment," while four said they had not undergone such a procedure. Six participants had health insurance, and three were uninsured. Eight participants had a regular health care provider.

FTM Youth

The FTM youth group included five participants, ranging in age from 16 to 25 with an average age of 21. Four participants identified as white and one as other. Two lived in Boston and three lived outside the Metro Boston area.

Three participants identified themselves as bisexual, one as "queer" and one as "none." Two participants were covered by their parents' insurance, one had MassHealth (Massachusetts' health care program for low-income individuals), one had insurance through school, and one participant was uninsured.

A more detailed description of how participants identified is presented in Table 1.

Disclosure of TG/TS Identity

In all four groups, participants discussed the difficulty of choosing when and how to disclose their transgender identity to a health care provider. Some of the MTF youth felt it was not always necessary to inform health care providers of their gender status: "What does being transgender have to do with my eyes?" In the FTM adult group, a participant stated, "That kind of information is on a need-to-know basis." He reported an incident in which he needed a wrist X-ray, and providers wrote in their notes that he was a transsexual "to educate others, because it was an educational institution. That was disrespectful." Another participant said he avoided disclosure by requesting that the providers start a brand new health chart at each visit: "I didn't want any evidence [of being female]." Other participants were adamant about the need for disclosure: "That's the first thing you do when you see a doctor," said one FTM adult. A feeling of trust in a primary care physi-

cian was a factor that encouraged disclosure. Some of the MTF youth, acknowledging the value of disclosure to the quality of their health care, said they actively seek out friendly, knowledgeable providers. One MTF adult said she called a clinic in advance to ask whether they were "TG/TS-friendly." Another MTF adult described a time when she "finally blurted it out" during an examination and found the provider was "very open" to her being a transsexual.

The lack of expectation of continuity in one's health care argued against disclosure, for some participants. One FTM adult said he had not disclosed his gender identity to his provider. He stated, *I'm afraid . . . I have had some bad experiences with health providers . . . so unless I'm convinced that I'm going to be with them a long time, I don't want to come out.*

Safety concerns can deter disclosure. One of the MTF youth described a nationally publicized 1995 incident in which a fire response team refused to treat an injured transgender individual, leading to her death. The MTF youth discussed concerns about safety upon disclosure outside of Massachusetts, which they perceived as progressive in terms of gender orientation and sexual preference. MTF youth also felt that even within Massachusetts, outside of

TABLE 1. Participants' Sex/Gender Identity; TG/TS Identity

MTF Adults	FTM Adults	MTF Youth	FTM Youth
Transgender; MTF	Male, Transsexual; FTM and Trans	Transgender; Female	Transsexual; Male
Transgender; MTF	Pre-transition transsexual; FTM	Transsexual/Female; Female	Transsexual; FTM
Transgender; MTF, Transgenderist	Male, Transsexual; FTM	Female; Female	Transgender; Male
Transsexual; MTF	Transsexual; FTM	Female; Female	Male; FTM
Transgender; MTF, post-operative	Transsexual; Male	Female; Female	Female, Transgender and Queer FTM; Trans and Queer
Transsexual; MTF	Male; FTM	Female; Female	
Transsexual; MTF	Male, Transsexual; FTM and Trans	Transsexual; Male to Female	
Transgender; MTF, Woman	Transsexual; FTM	Female; Male to Female	
	Transsexual; FTM and Male	Other; Male to Female	
	Male; Male		
	Transsexual; Trans and Male		
	Transsexual; FTM		

the urban center of Boston, a sense of trans community was unlikely and disclosure less safe. In all groups, participants illuminated the real risks of disclosure in terms of health care coverage.

An FTM youth participant said,

> ... (A)t best, the doctor will treat me but report me in my medical records, which in turn will 'out' me to an insurance company that will in turn deny me health coverage for anything they say is related to me being trans.

In each of the groups, some participants said that a difficult component of disclosure was the need to inform health care providers how to refer properly to the gender of a TG/TS individual. In the MTF adult group, one participant described her anger when a provider was unwilling to refer to her as "she," and continued referring to her as "he," despite repeated requests.

Health Issues

Participants identified a variety of health issues. In all groups, participants revealed their need for medical and psychological services common to the general population. In addition, participants described service needs particular to TG/TS individuals, mainly hormone treatments and sex reassignment surgery (SRS); and mental health and substance abuse treatment tailored to TG/TS clients.

Across all groups, participants identified needs for primary/general medical care, dentistry and mental health/substance abuse treatment. The adult MTF group saw substance abuse treatment and HIV/AIDS care as key; one MTF participant, a former prostitute, noted the deaths of 15 TG/TS friends, related to violence, substance abuse, or HIV/AIDS.

Both MTF groups considered endocrinology and hormone therapy to be major health issues. The MTF adult group said that endocrinology, mental health and primary care were their most important health care needs, but also mentioned hepatitis treatment, psychopharmacology (medicines used to treat mental health conditions), and ophthalmology (eye care beyond corrective lenses). The MTF youth reported usage of a wide variety of health services, including primary care, mental health, dentistry, electrolysis, plastic surgery and silicone injections.

Both of the adult groups mentioned sex reassignment surgery (SRS) as important. The MTF adult group discussed related needs, ranging from information resources about SRS to follow-up gynecological care. The FTM youth participants cited inadequate provider education on FTM adolescent health issues. Participants in the FTM youth group mentioned their need for general/primary health care, gynecology, hormone therapy, endocrinology, dermatology, dental care, substance abuse treatment and mental health support, including treatment for depression and anorexia.

Hormone Therapy

Within each group, participants comprised a wide range of personal experience with hormone therapy and SRS. For example, in the FTM adult group, several participants said they had undergone surgery to reconstruct their bodies; one person said he did not want to take hormones or modify his body through surgery. Participants who had undergone or wished to undergo these therapies described a variety of hurdles to obtaining desired services. In the MTF adult group, discussion focused on how participants used hormones and their concerns about the long-term medical effects of hormone therapy. Many participants in the MTF adult group said they do take or have taken hormones without medical supervision; one participant said she had increased her own dosage of hormones in order to speed her transformation. Another participant reported a stroke, leg swelling and kidney damage that she believes might be due to prolonged use of hormones.

In the MTF youth group, participants discussed the amount of therapy and exams required in order to obtain hormone therapy: "Health care providers want too much from you to give you so little." Even at a Boston clinic known to welcome TG/TS people, one MTF participant stated that hormone therapy only was offered due to repeated requests from clients. Participants agreed that self-advocacy was critical to obtaining hormone therapy, as well as other health care. One MTF youth cited obstacles to obtaining hormone therapy while she was in the care of a state run agency. "[The agency] is so vicious towards transsexuals." This participant stated that she was able to obtain hormone therapy more easily in prison than through this public agency.

In the MTF youth group, of seven participants using hormones, several reported obtaining their hormones illegally and one participant said she obtained prescriptions another way: *I don't want to wait around six months so someone could tell me, 'you are what you say you are.' I started calling in prescriptions under my father's name and it worked.*

Some in the MTF youth group said they had obtained hormones from friends, due to a lack of other options. Several participants in the MTF youth group believed that inconsistent provider implementation of standards for TG/TS health care limits their access to hormone therapy. The group shared a perception that providers are moving toward standards, signifying a readiness to address the needs of TG/TS clients. However, although the standards may recommend prescription of hormones, participants anticipated that access to hormones would come slowly because standards are not universally acknowledged or applied. An MTF youth participant said that at one health center, providers told her that decisions regarding a hormone prescription for her were "on hold" while the agency established therapeutic guidelines. Another participant, in an effort to obtain hormone therapy, showed her practitioner the TG/TS health care standards published by the Harry Benjamin International Gender Dysphoria Association, Inc. (HBIGDA), the professional organization devoted to the understanding and treatment of gender identity disorders, and creators of the internationally accepted guidelines on treatment; until then, the practitioner had been unaware of these standards (HBIGDA, 2001).

Participants in the FTM adult group who had not used hormone or SRS therapies described problems related to providers' ignorance about TG/TS conditions:

> *I'm not interested in medically transitioning, but I want the recognition of masculinity in terms of getting called by male pronouns . . . it's not like I need*

access to immediate hormones and surgery, but I need the respect and people to know that I am uncomfortable with a lot of parts of my body.

Mental Health Issues

In the area of mental health, many participants reported distressing experiences. In the FTM adult group, participants said they often have to educate therapists on transgender issues. One participant reported that a therapist asked him, "Why didn't you just stay a woman?" Another participant stated that a mental health provider said to him, "You're just a different kind of woman"; the participant described feeling hurt and insulted by this comment: "If I could've lived as a 'different kind of woman' it would've been a lot easier."

In the MTF youth group, participants stated that in some instances, mental health consultations are only sought to satisfy a prerequisite for obtaining hormones. Several MTF youth described their disappointments with the mental health care they had received, mentioning therapists' lack of experience with trans people; therapists' lack of experience with TG/TS youth; overcharging by therapists; and being "bumped between therapists" at an agency. The adult MTF group presented a different perspective on mental health and hormones. The majority of participants in the MTF adult group said they currently were seeing a mental health practitioner, in some cases due to mood swings caused by hormone therapy. Other mental health problems reported by MTF participants included depression, suicidal feelings, anorexia, difficulty in decision-making regarding SRS, and treatment for post-traumatic stress disorder after being raped.

When mental health needs include treatment for substance abuse, TG/TS people face special barriers, according to participants. Many saw the mental health component of substance abuse treatment as insensitive to and ineffective with the particular issues of trans people. One MTF adult said that during her substance abuse rehabilitation in a hospital, providers avoided discussing gender issues, "which is ironic, as [gender issues] had everything to do with it." An FTM adult said that finding a therapist was difficult when he began recovery from substance abuse, because therapists refused to help him deal simultaneously with his substance abuse and gender issues: "[I was told], 'Deal with your substance abuse, and then come back.'"

Quality and Standards of Care

All groups were guided to establish definitions of quality health care and evaluate the quality of care they have received. In all four groups, participants agreed that quality health care hinged on providers' willingness to listen, learn, and allocate time to discuss conditions and issues unique to TG/TS people. "It's more than just reading your chart," said one MTF youth participant. Some participants said that the quality of care is greatly helped by access to continuity of providers and consistency in policies for health care. In all groups, participants felt that medical providers' ignorance compromised the quality of care.

In the FTM adult group, one participant said that a provider who is not sure what "transgender" means ought to let the client know: "It is unethical for them not to do that. . . . We're supposed to be giving informed consent to be treated. So we are entitled to know, reasonably, if they have any experience [with transgender issues]."

In the MTF youth group, participants raised the point that a health care experience included not just one's interaction with a provider, but also her interactions with receptionists and other staff during the medical visit. An FTM adult echoed this perception: "I think it is . . . important for the support staff to be comfortable, because they are the gatekeepers."

FTM youth said they frequently encountered verbal abuse and condescension from frontline health care staff such as receptionists: "I can't even make it through the front door without staff staring at me, laughing at me or whispering about my gender presentation." In the FTM youth group, all participants agreed that they did not feel safe receiving health care; one described his health care experience as "traumatizing."

Provider acceptance of one's gender self-identification was a key aspect of quality health care. An FTM adult said that it made him uncomfortable when his provider "kept referring to me as 'people like you.'" One FTM youth found experiences with gynecological care especially upsetting: "There is a lack of sensitivity when I have to have a gynecological examination . . . The doctor was not sensitive to the fact that I experience myself as male and that this experience was overwhelming for me." Said one FTM adult, "I think for me it is respect and a willingness to respect your pronoun. I found that to be a huge problem. As somebody that hasn't done any body alterations, it's hard for people to switch pronouns and accept the pronoun [that I prefer]."

The adult FTM group agreed that the quality of health care was enhanced when it was possible to see the same individual provider at each health care visit: "There are residents (who) are interested, but if I impart a piece of information to one, and . . . see a different resident the next time, it doesn't give me any continuity and I have to explain my whole story over again."

In the MTF youth group, there was discussion about a provider that is sensitive to TG/TS health issues, but whose quality of care was compromised by a protracted process of creating agency-specific standards of care concerning eligibility for hormone use and/or other medical procedures (no further clarification was given regarding the employment of the HBIGDA standards of care). One participant in the group said that her hormone treatments were delayed for several months while a policy was established regarding the type of treatment she needed.

Accessing Health Care

Access to health care had two components: (1) locating providers who were knowledgeable about transgender health issues and comfortable with TG/TS people, and (2) securing and paying for specific needed services.

In all groups, participant statements suggested that discomfort in the health care system had the potential to limit their access to care at any point along the continuum from seeking care to obtaining and paying for it. For example, FTM adult participants said "For ten years I didn't go to a doctor at all," and "I didn't go to a dentist because I knew she wouldn't be comfortable." Another FTM adult said he would only access care if he were very ill: "I just don't want to be in a medical environment and be vulnerable to all the [difficulties] we've been talking about."

A lack of trust in providers hindered some participants' access to HIV testing. One participant in the FTM adult group said he was reluctant to describe his sex life to a provider, and therefore "would not talk to one of these doctors about safe sex." In the same group, one participant said he was reluctant to be tested for HIV, because of the questions it might spark from a doctor.

Locating Knowledgeable Providers

While some participants used Health Maintenance Organizations (HMOs), teaching hospitals and community health centers to locate and access services, a variety of alternative means were mentioned. For example, adult FTM participants mentioned the Internet, networking in the trans community, friends, coworkers, and a partner as resources for locating health care providers.

Beyond the basic standard that providers be educated about trans issues and conditions, participants discussed several specific issues regarding provider setting. Some participants sought gay-identified clinics, while others avoided them. An FTM adult who has a child mentioned the difficulty of finding a family health care setting where providers were comfortable with his being a parent. Another FTM adult said, "I go someplace where they see a lot of us [TG/TS people] so if I need to see somebody in a related area [I feel more comfortable]." In the MTF youth group, a participant who did not live in an urban area said that she had found appropriate providers in Boston, but "I have to come here every time I need to see someone. It is really inconvenient." In the FTM adult group, participants discussed the greater difficulty in accessing quality care for people living farther from a city, "people who are less socially sophisticated, or people who speak different languages."

Referrals to other health care practitioners were not always experienced as safe. One FTM adult described what happened when he followed up on a referral for surgery:

I assumed that since I was at [a trans-friendly medical center] it would be fine, and I had [had] other surgery there that was absolutely wonderful . . . He asked about the scars on my chest [from reconstructive surgery], and when I told him what they were, his mouth dropped open and bounced off the floor, and he said, 'What are you talking about?' . . . That was it. I was packed up and sent away.

A similar anecdote was told by an FTM youth:

I was referred to a specialist and my doctor never told the specialist about my condition and the fact that I was on hormones . . . the specialist was harsh with me and treated me like I had mental health problems stemming from the fact that I was transgender.

The FTM youth group discussed a lack of referral resources available from providers. One participant said that his local mental health provider's limited references (i.e., the network of available providers as determined by his health insurance) kept him "locked" into one circle of providers.

All groups discussed resources outside the conventional health care system that can provide information and support for TG/TS people. In the FTM adult group, one participant said, "We have to be our own physicians in that we have to interact with other people going through the same thing and find out what [they] are doing." For participants in the FTM youth group, the Internet was a crucial resource, offering a safe forum for finding current, relevant health information in both Web sites and chat rooms. In the MTF adult group, many had used the Internet to locate health care information, and one participant said she had used it to find the surgeon in Europe who performed her SRS surgery.

Participants in all groups said that regardless of their ability to find appropriate health care providers, securing access to needed health care still presented problems. "I was actually turned away [from an emergency room] because the doctor said he did not treat people like me," said one FTM youth.

Securing and Paying for Needed Services

Participants' comments reflected that the trans population shares the challenges that face the general population in securing health insurance. One MTF youth said insurance is difficult "to come by if a person is not in school, or does not have a job that includes insurance." Medical needs and concerns specific to being trans appear to make the journey toward health insurance especially challenging. One FTM adult reported that TG/TS people reverse the typical process of finding health care: "We choose the doctor first, and then the insurance. And that can be a huge barrier to getting care."

In all groups, participants expressed fear of disclosing their trans identity to insurers, for fear of facing exclusions in or loss of their health care coverage. In the FTM youth group, a participant said, "Even when I do work and pay for an HMO [Health Maintenance Organization], they don't cover my health care cost because I have identified as transgender." One FTM adult said that his health insurance plan specifically excludes transsexual surgery, while another said he did not know what his insurance covered: "I'm almost afraid to raise the issue. I haven't told my employer, so I'm not sure what the hell I'm entitled to."

One FTM adult, after he had enrolled in an insurance plan, did not want to inform the insurance company that he was TG/TS: "It wasn't just finding a primary care physician . . . there were extra steps I had to take [to ensure quality care]. I had to say, 'Please don't put anything in your records at this time.'" Another FTM adult wanted to go outside of a health care plan for mental health treatment:

> . . . but I was afraid that if I put down the reason I wanted out-of-network coverage, it would flag my being a transsexual and then I might lose my coverage for endocrinology and hormone therapy. So I withdrew it and opted to pay out of pocket.

In the MTF youth group, participants who had health insurance said that basic services were covered, but not endocrinology or hormone therapy. The MTF adult group's statements corroborated that the lack of coverage for hormone therapy and/or SRS by insurance plans,

Social Security Disability Insurance (SSDI–federally-funded insurance for disabled workers), or Medicaid (federally-funded, state-run insurance for low income individuals) is a barrier to accessing these services.

In the FTM youth group, participants discussed ways to circumvent the policies of health insurers in order to obtain services. Participants said that some providers will report falsely that a patient requires therapy for a hormone imbalance, to ensure that insurance will cover the costs of hormones. An FTM adult said, "We don't have to just be experts on transsexuality; we have to be experts on the health care system." Another FTM adult said, "We have to finesse the system because most things aren't covered by insurance." Like the general population, trans people are vulnerable to limits that provider systems place on the amount and duration of treatment. In the MTF adult group, participants agreed that HMO limits on mental health counseling presented a hardship.

At the simple level of paperwork, standard forms can be barriers to health care for trans individuals. The MTF youth group discussed the legality of checking "male" or "female" based on one's self-described gender identity; one participant said, "There is no box for me, so as far as I'm concerned [checking my self-described gender] is not false." However, there is a lingering concern that insurers will reject claims by trans individuals if they fraudulently identify their gender.

Relationships with Health Care Providers

Trust in an individual provider and the anticipation of being listened to were the key attributes that participants identified for a positive relationship with health care systems and providers. However, most of the experiences described by participants illustrated a climate where, based on past experiences, TG/TS people mistrust providers and expect not to be listened to in a health care setting.

In all groups, participants said they had encountered humiliating treatment from providers and outright refusal to provide services. One MTF adult said that when a provider discovered her transsexuality, the provider refused to treat her and commented that she should 'see a veterinarian' as a medical doctor was 'a doctor for people.' In the FTM adult group, one participant, who has a child, described an obstetrics/gynecology provider's reaction to his disclosure that he was transgender: " The change was remarkable." The participant stated that after disclosure, the provider felt that his parenting was inappropriate and questioned why he wanted both ob/gyn care and hormones–evidence of ignorance about transgender issues, according to the participant.

In the FTM youth group, participants discussed a lack of sensitivity and awareness on the part of providers; said one participant, "They do not listen when I tell them that I have body issues and that I do not relate to my body as female." Another FTM youth said that a doctor caused him to leave the office in tears by suggesting a birth control prescription to address his complaint of gender dysphoria: "We are being penalized for being truthful about ourselves by both doctors and health insurance companies."

At times, unnecessary attention to their trans identity made participants uncomfortable with providers. Participants in the FTM youth group stated that providers focused on their gender identity despite its irrelevance to the reason for the medical visit, such as flu symptoms.

The FTM adult group agreed that a provider's willingness to listen was the key to a good relationship:

> It's really important that you have a physician or a nurse who will listen to what our concerns are . . . because it's not the average concern.

and,

> We have knowledge that if they listen to us . . . and take that as a starting place, then they're a lot further ahead than if they just treat us all as if we're all the same.

In the MTF youth group, one participant shared this belief, saying that a good provider was someone who "might not have all the answers, but who is willing to listen."

In the FTM adult group, some participants said they more quickly trust a nurse than a doctor:

> I almost immediately trust a nurse. It's like they're in the trenches. They have a different demeanor with you than the doctor does.

Some FTM adult participants said they try to help educate providers, but often encounter the provider's lack of interest in and time for listening. In the FTM adult group, a participant said he offers educational videotapes to providers, in order to educate them about TG/TS issues. He stated,

> Some will watch it to see what we're about, and others will take it and not even look at it, and not even be interested . . . To me, how interested are they in our concerns and needs if they aren't interested in spending . . . half an hour to research what we might be about?

In one case, cancellations by other patients gave one physician the time to be receptive to a FTM adult participant:

> The doctor spent an hour and a half with me, and after a year of fighting with [various providers], I finally had someone here who listened. And he agreed with my self-treatment and my self-assessment . . . but I don't know if that would've happened if the weather had been better. I would have had 15 minutes and that would have been the end of it.

Another FTM adult participant noted that not all providers are willing to listen and learn from patients: "When you have information that your primary care provider doesn't, sometimes they resent that."

In mental health units, detox centers or shelters, most of the FTM youth said they do not feel safe or accommodated: "It tends to be the staff that has more problems with me being transgender than the other clients or patients [have]." In general, this group felt that physicians and mental health providers do not want to treat FTM youth: "If they wanted to provide us services, they would treat us like human beings instead of freaks"; "I have to be deathly sick before I go to a doctor."

Some participants had preferences as to the gender of their provider. In the MTF adult group, most participants said they felt more comfortable with a female provider, although one said: "There are some males that are good . . . it depends on the person." The reasons cited for preferring a female provider included participants' feeling that it was easier to communicate with a female, as well as that they were more comfortable being examined or touched by a female, due to the gynecological and hormonal aspects of the care they required. One FTM adult participant said that gender didn't matter, "as long as they are respectful, knowledgeable, and willing to listen to what my issues are." "I am looking for a doctor who will treat me like a human being with feelings," said one FTM youth participant.

Participants' Recommendations

All groups made specific recommendations to improve health care access and quality of services for TG/TS people. The FTM adult group stressed that providers should be made aware of what transgender is and its implications for a person's health and health care.

> I think they have a responsibility to be educated about us before we walk in there. It's important that they listen while we're there, but it's important that they have some prior knowledge that's out there and available.

In addition, in order to feel comfortable and satisfied with their health care, the FTM adults wanted assurance that providers who are educated about TG/TS issues also are competent practitioners: "It's important that a person not only has a sense of who . . . works with transgendered people, but also works well and is respected as a professional."

The FTM youth developed these priorities for medical care: a safe provider environment that (1) can provide health care with respect to being TG/TS, (2) is educated on transgender issues, and (3) provides a way to pay for its services.

The MTF youth group agreed that education and training of staff–including providers, administrators, and reception staff–would help agencies develop competence in providing care to trans people. Participants suggested that providers and agencies create and familiarize themselves with reasonable policies and standards so that all parties involved in TG/TS health care can share the same expectations about care and procedures. Additionally, one MTF youth participant recommended that each client be treated as an individual: "We might have some things in common, but we're not all the same."

Participants in several groups recommended that providers create and use more inclusive intake forms to incorporate TG/TS individuals, either by letting individuals self-identify their gender or, as the MTF youth group suggested, "adding an extra box." In the MTF youth group, one participant urged self-education and self-advocacy for TG/TS people to ensure their ability to obtain proper health care. The group agreed that access to the Internet and knowledge of how to use it would be very helpful to clients (as well as providers) for education and networking for health care information and support. The MTF adult group asked for more research into prolonged use of hormones, and application of technology, such as MRI (Magnetic Resonance Imaging) scanning of individuals for blood clots that hormones may cause. The MTF adults also asked that clinics that serve a TG/TS population offer full coverage for hormone therapy and SRS. They added that visible representation of trans individuals on staff and in provider publications would make TG/TS clients more comfortable in a health care provider setting.

DISCUSSION

This study set out to investigate a premise that in accessing even the most basic health care, trans people interact with health care systems that may not be prepared and providers who may not be educated to address their needs and concerns ("Health Concerns . . . ," 1997; Haynes, 1998). A further premise of this study was that most providers and systems neither anticipate nor fund particular services that TG/TS individuals require. The focus group findings corroborated these premises, and revealed a variety of barriers for trans individuals seeking health care.

Focus group participants offered diverse examples of the barriers to health care that they encountered. Some were subtle and some were blatant. The barriers ranged from refusal to treat to inappropriate intake forms for a trans person to the lack of insurance coverage for sex reassignment treatments and procedures under the current health care system.

In fact, many health insurers do limit health care for trans individuals by excluding sexual reassignment surgery and/or hormones from coverage (Tufts Health Plan, 1998; Oxford Health Plans, 2003). For example, one insurance policy excludes any *procedure or treatment designed to alter the physical characteristics of a Member from the Member's biological sex to those of the opposite sex, regardless of any diagnosis of gender role or psychosexual orientation problems* (Oxford Health Plans, 2003).

Such policy restrictions are exacerbated by a general lack of standards across the provider world for treating trans-related conditions. Thus, transgendered and transsexual individuals are correct that disclosing their gender identity may lead to loss of coverage. Participant statements in the focus groups suggest that many trans people do indeed approach full disclosure with trepidation, much as gay and lesbian individuals may fear "coming out" to their health care providers ("Access and Use of Health Services . . . ," 1997).

As with most qualitative studies, this investigation yielded much information that indicates areas of concern, yet leaves much to be quantified and verified by future studies (see "Recommendations," below). One caveat for any further study of health care access among TG/TS people–whether qualitative or quantitative–is that much work still needs to be done in terms of effectively categorizing people who identify as transsexual or transgender. In this study, the difficulty of assigning individuals to an appropriate group presented methodological challenges and essentially limited the scope and power of the study.

The study limited itself by convening focus groups of transgendered or transsexual people who self-identified as transitioning from male-to-female or female-to-male. The study was unlikely to reveal the unique health care issues and barriers that may exist for self-identified nongendered (not identifying with either male or female, and often preferring to use pronouns tied to neither gender, such as "zie" or "zir") people or others who do not identify with the concept of "transitioning" as an aspect of their gender. Additionally, the fact that all participants identified with some aspect of "trans" terminology, these groups still comprised many nuances of TG/TS identity. Within the groups, it was difficult to find patterns in participants' experiences because individuals' identities could not be categorized accurately enough for comparisons.

Participant statements in all four groups revealed significant emotional pain and in some cases outright fear when using the health care system. Such discomfort, unbalanced by positive experiences, clearly indicates a gap in health care access for TG/TS individuals. The obvious step forward is to work toward a situation where trans individuals can count on no less of a welcome from their health care providers than other consumers receive (see "Recommendations").

The transgender population does not lend itself easily to conventional sociological methods of study. Two types of difficulties were identified in undertaking this study: group dynamics and evolving language.

In each group, the fact that many participants and the facilitators knew one another most likely affected the nature of the group's discussion. In the two adult groups, the facilitator had recruited the participants and was on a first-name basis with most of them. The familiarity within the groups may reflect the size of the trans community in Greater Boston. The familiarity among individuals in the groups may have inhibited participants from talking about their current personal issues, especially regarding sensitive subjects such as sexual behavior and drug use.

In the MTF adult group, stories about the past, rather than current situations, were more generally shared. Participants talked about drug use and sexual experience in the TG/TS community, although rarely talking specifically about themselves. Similarly, participants in the adult FTM group talked about social issues within their community, but spoke less about their own sexual and drug issues. In one exception, one FTM adult who was gay-identified did talk about having unprotected sex.

In the youth MTF group, discussion did not touch upon personal sexual behaviors or drug use. Frank discussion of these topics may have been inhibited by the presence of the recruiter (a friend to many participants); a male note taker from JSI staff; and a facilitator known to many youth in the community. After the group disbanded, the recruiter and the facilitator mentioned that some participants had downplayed their personal problems; the facilitator said she knew this from working with these youth and being privy to their lives.

The discussions in all four focus groups demonstrate the important fact that the language for describing TG/TS people and issues is not fixed, but evolving. Medical science, social construct, and personal experience each contribute to the terms that exist, and the ways people use and understand them.

Although we expected to gather straightforward information about participants' self-identifications with the screening instrument, these expectations were confounded by responses.

Participants were asked to describe themselves three different ways:

1. What is your sex or gender? (Response categories were Transgender, Transsexual, Male, Female, and Other with space for write-in)
2. What is your transsexual/transgender identity? (Response categories were Male to Female, Female to Male, Trans, Male, Female, and Other with space for write-in)
3. What is your sexual orientation? (Response categories were Heterosexual, Gay, Lesbian, Bisexual, Heterosexual, and Other with space for write-in)

The survey instrument allowed respondents freedom to choose more than one identification word in each question. Further, many individuals handwrote additional choices for the second two questions.

Participants varied widely in their self-identification. For example, while one individual in a group might indicate a self-identification of both transsexual and transgender, another might reject the former term and select the latter. In the MTF adult group, three people who in the screening instrument identified as transsexual

or female, later in conversation expressed strong dislike of the term "transgender." By contrast, in both youth groups, a larger proportion of participants embraced the term transgender. The apparent preference for the term "transgender" over "transsexual" among younger participants may reflect differences in both social and physical attributes among individuals, or it may indeed reflect changing cultural norms around language over time. In any case, this observation suggests a starting point for studying the use and meaning of language among TG/TS people.

RECOMMENDATIONS

An established vocabulary for trans people and issues is needed to increase dialogue in the health care realm. Even the participants in this study had difficulty settling on words to describe and discuss themselves. Prior to the establishment of language that providers can use to discuss and address TG/TS clients respectfully and helpfully, the existing language must be studied to capture the terms and definitions most widely accepted. Attention to the language for trans people and conditions will contribute to comfortable self-identification for TG/TS people as well as dissemination of appropriate language to providers, agencies and others who address their health care needs.

Fitting people into boxes is necessary for meaningful sociological study, however, with this population, categorization proves a big challenge. Metaphorically as well as literally speaking, there is no standardized form for this cohort. In further studies of this nature, we recommend detailed attention to the language used in both a screening instrument and in questions for the groups' discussion. The findings of this study also suggest a need for opportunities for TG/TS people to share with health care providers appropriate language that fits and describes their many, diverse, unique identities.

In order for the health care system to better serve trans people, it must not only find ways to listen better to these consumers, but must initiate dialogue about their identities, concerns, and specific health care needs.

This study undertook to gather opinions and information from four focus groups, in order to explore the following questions:

- What gaps in health care exist for TG/TS individuals, and how can they be filled?

- What can providers and agencies do to make a TG/TS individual feel, and be, welcome and well cared for?
- What resources are available to providers, agencies, and consumers to facilitate high quality health care for trans people?

Across the four focus groups, a constant theme was a perception of vast provider ignorance of trans people and concerns. From the level of health care systems down to individual providers and frontline staff, TG/TS people reported provider unawareness of, disrespect toward, and outright refusal of treatment for their health needs, both basic and trans-related. Many of the health care gaps that participants experienced stem from the discomfort they reported on initial contact with a health care system. Clearly, an immediate need exists to reduce the "frontline" barrier to basic health care that many trans people reported in this study. A primary recommendation would embrace any activities to increase provider awareness of trans people and issues and to reinforce provider understanding of the basic right of all human beings to basic health care services.

This recommendation is substantiated by a recent policy statement from the American Public Health Association (APHA), which urges researchers and health care workers to categorize transgender individuals as male-to-female, female-to-male or other as appropriate, and *not conflate them with gay men or lesbians (unless as appropriate to an individual's sexual orientation in their preferred gender) as well as acknowledging the variation that exists among trans individuals* (American Public Health Association, 1999).

The APHA report also corroborates another recommendation: that a targeted effort is needed to establish and deliver to health care providers information about appropriate language pertaining to transsexual and transgender people, conditions and procedures. The APHA report reminds the provider community to "refer to them [trans individuals] as the gender with which they identify," and "be sensitive to the lives of transgendered individuals and treat them with dignity and respect." We, too, believe that a targeted effort is needed to remind providers, especially "frontlines" personnel, to affirm each patient's human dignity by holding

assumptions in check, and listening and responding to the patient's self-description of identity and self-assessment of health care need.

A further step would encourage providers to examine or develop, and then adopt, standards for transgender/transsexual health care. TG/TS people reported that they are uncertain as to what services are available, and therefore may be tempted to find illegal means to procure and/or finance particular services (especially SRS and hormone therapy). Besides being unlawful, such resourcefulness may put consumers in medical danger, as much needs to be learned about safe and proper hormone dosage. In pursuit of appropriate provider standards for trans-related medical care, clinical research is needed into the long-range affects of prolonged use of hormones.

Finally, it is recommended that a deeper study of the interaction between trans people and the health care system take place. In addition to further qualitative exploration, we recommend a quantitative study to map more precisely the health care gaps for TG/TS people and to assess in more depth the numbers, diversity and geographical clustering of trans individuals throughout Massachusetts. Such a study might include employment, socioeconomic status, age, and specific health care coverage of self-identified TG/TS participants. Any information-gathering effort that can help determine the characteristics and needs of a trans community and/or its sub-communities will help open provider arms and close the health care gap.

REFERENCES CITED

Access and Use of Health Services by Lesbians and Gay Men in the Greater Boston Area: An Exploratory Study (1997). Prepared by John Snow, Inc.

American Public Health Association (1999). Policy Statements Adopted by the Governing Council of the American Public Health Association.

Bakker, A., Kesteren, P.J.M. van Gooren, L.J.G., & Bezemer, P.D. (1993). The prevalence of transsexualism in the Netherlands. Acta Psychiatr Scand, 87, 237-238.

Clements K., Wilkinson W., Kitano K., Ph.D., Marx R., Ph.D. (1999) HIV Prevention and Health Service

Needs of the Transgender Community in San Francisco. IJT 3,1+2. Available online at http://www.symposion.com/ijt/hiv_risk/clements.htm.

Clements, K. (1999). The Transgender Community Health Project: Descriptive Results. Prepared for the San Francisco Department of Public Health.

Harry Benjamin International Gender Dysphoria Association, Inc. (2001). Standards of Care, Version Six. Available online at http://www.hbigda.org/soc.cfm.

Haynes, R. (1998). Towards Healthier Transgender Youth. Crossroads. Winter, pp. 14-15.

Health Concerns of the Gay, Lesbian, Bisexual, and Transgender Community (2nd ed.) (1997). Prepared by The Medical Foundation.

Mason, T., Connors, M., Kammerer, C. (1995). Transgenders and HIV Risks: Needs Assessment. Prepared for the Massachusetts Department of Public Health, HIV/AIDS Bureau. Gender Identity Support Services for Transgenders (GISST).

Oxford Health Plans (October 2003), Oxford HMO/Freedom Network Plan. Section V: Exclusions and Limitations.

Tufts Health Plan, Point of Service Plan (October 1998). Exclusions and Limitations.

Identifying Training Needs of Health-Care Providers Related to Treatment and Care of Transgendered Patients: A Qualitative Needs Assessment Conducted in New England

Samuel Lurie

SUMMARY. The Transgender Training Project of the New England AIDS Education and Training Center has been providing training on transgender-related issues to health-care providers in the New England region since 1999, having trained nearly 600 providers in that time. The Transgender Training Project embarked on a study during the 2001-2002 grant year to interview providers of HIV-related care and advocacy on their knowledge and experience with working with transgendered people and to assess training needs to increase their effectiveness with transgendered clients.

The methodology consisted of face-to-face interviews with 13 providers of HIV treatment and care who are affiliated with the New England AIDS Education and Training Center network to discuss clinical challenges in working with transgendered people.

In this exploratory study, we found that providers had:

1. Desire to treat transgendered patients respectfully but admitted discomfort and lack of tools for specific interviewing/assessments.
2. Experience with a range of transgendered patients, but lack of information on distinctions among transgendered experiences.

Samuel Lurie is Principle Investigator, Transgender Training Project of the New England AIDS Education and Training Center (Website: *www.tgtrain.org*; E-mail: slurie@gmavt.net).

Khady Ndao-Bromblay, PharmD, offered invaluable guidance in the development of the questions and methodology; Terry Ruefli, PhD, executive director of the New York Harm Reduction Educators Inc., and Jackie Weinstock, PhD, of the University of Vermont both generously shared insight and expertise in developing the Findings categories. Walter Bockting, PhD, provided thorough and insightful editing of the final article. The author is also indebted to researchers who shared their work: Kristin Clements-Nolle, MPH; Emelia Lombardi, PhD; Gretchen Kenagy, PhD; Walter Bockting, PhD, and Carrie Davis, all generously shared both published and background material with the author and helped to inform and shape the tone of this project. The author also received assistance from several people working at clinics–Katie Douglass, MSW, at the Callen-Lorde Health Center in New York; Mary Monihan, NP, at the Tom Waddell Health Center in San Francisco; and Diego Sanchez of the TransHealth Education Program at JRI in Boston all shared information on their protocols, clinic experiences and community responses to their work. Finally, the author is grateful to the health-care providers who reviewed early versions of the interview questions, those who referred other colleagues and, of course, those who agreed to be interviewed. Their willingness to share their time and expertise, and to honestly reflect on real challenges, made this project possible.

This research was funded by the New England AIDS Education and Training Center, U.S. Department of Health and Human Services, Health Resources and Services Administration, Federal Grant Number NEAETC FY 2001-2001–5 H4A HA 00013-03.

[Haworth co-indexing entry note]: "Identifying Training Needs of Health-Care Providers Related to Treatment and Care of Transgendered Patients: A Qualitative Needs Assessment Conducted in New England." Lurie, Samuel. Co-published simultaneously in *International Journal of Transgenderism* (The Haworth Medical Press, an imprint of The Haworth Press, Inc.) Vol. 8, No. 2/3, 2005, pp. 93-112; and: *Transgender Health and HIV Prevention: Needs Assessment Studies from Transgender Communities Across the United States* (ed: Walter Bockting, and Eric Avery) The Haworth Medical Press, an imprint of The Haworth Press, Inc., 2005, pp. 93-112. Single or multiple copies of this article are available for a fee from The Haworth Document Delivery Service [1-800-HAWORTH, 9:00 a.m. - 5:00 p.m. (EST). E-mail address: docdelivery@haworthpress.com].

3. Restrictions based on time constraints that create an overarching barrier in building trusting relationships with clients, and trusting relationships are integral to quality care.
4. Concern and frustration with lack of information, studies and research.
5. Concern and frustration with lack of treatment guidelines, (or ability to access them), referral contacts and ways to advocate for transgender clients.
6. Belief that training by transgendered people themselves was an essential teaching element.

These results point to the need for the development and dissemination of specific training materials and resources for health-care providers serving transgendered people living with or at risk for HIV. *[Article copies available for a fee from The Haworth Document Delivery Service: 1-800-HAWORTH. E-mail address: <docdelivery@haworthpress.com> Website: <http://www.HaworthPress.com> © 2005 by The Haworth Press, Inc. All rights reserved.]*

KEYWORDS. Transgender, training needs, health care, HIV/AIDS

INTRODUCTION

With studies spanning back a decade, HIV prevention and treatment providers have been seeing alarming signs of the impact of HIV on transgendered people. Prevalence studies have shown strikingly high rates of HIV among transgendered populations. Studies of transgendered sex workers have found 68% in a study in Atlanta (Elifson, 1994) and a 1998 study in San Francisco–the largest scale study to date–some of the starkest evidence was gathered: 35% of the group was HIV positive and 63% of African-American male-to-female subgroup were found to be HIV positive (Clements-Nolle et al., 2001). Of this, many learned of their status by being tested as part of the study itself.

A number of findings have been consistent and telling as members of the transgendered community have been surveyed in community-based needs assessments. Highly marginalized lives mix with other issues such as poverty, racism, violence, lack of housing and employment options and damaging or discouraging experiences with medical providers put transgendered people at high risk for HIV and make it difficult for transgendered people to obtain respectful, quality care.

A primary finding of these needs assessments is that health care providers lack basic knowledge and need to be trained on working with transgendered people. Participants in focus groups and interviews have reported experiences of being refused care, mistreated, harassed and ridiculed by providers (Clements,

1998; Elifson, 1993; Bockting, 1998; McGowan, 1999; Kammerer, 1995; Xavier, 2000; GLBT Health Access, 2000; Kenagy, 2002). Transgendered people have said that negative experiences with providers, including HIV test counselors, prevent them from seeking HIV testing (GLBT Health Access, 2000).

In related studies, HIV-positive participants have stated that they receive confusing messages from medical providers and that they need more information about hormone therapy and gender reassignment surgery to make informed decisions (Bockting, 1998; Clements-Nolle, 1999). Indeed, very little information is readily available for providers to assist patients in making informed decisions and much of the knowledge is developing in practices with high numbers of HIV-positive transgendered people. Even providers in those settings have little or no training and are experiencing a steep learning curve as they work with patients for whom there is little clinical research to guide the way.

The word "transgender" is generally used as an umbrella term for a wide range of people who do not fit neatly into traditional societal views of male and female, man and woman. One way of looking at how society constructs language and concepts around gender is to refer to our dominant cultural paradigm as "bi-gendered," that is, only two genders are commonly recognized. Transgender experience encompasses a range of people who experience their own identity, or express that identity to the outside world, in ways that broaden the boundaries of a two-gender system. Some transgendered people, however, believe perfectly well in the two-gender system, and feel they were simply assigned the wrong gender at birth. "Transsexual" is generally used to distinguish those who desire to live full-time in the gender role different than the one assigned at birth, and who take or plan to take hormonal and/or surgical interventions to have their bodies better fit that role. (Further, transexual spelled with one 's' is the preferred community spelling; whereas two s's, transsexual, is the more common medical community spelling. The former spelling connotes community and identity whereas the latter focuses more on a medical model based on a bi-gender construct) (Bockting, 1997).

Male-to-female (MTF) is the common term for those born biologically male who express or feel their gender in more feminine ways; and female-to-male (FTM) is used for those born biologically female who express or experience their gender in more masculine ways. Both constitute spectrums, or continuums, with a range of experience, expressions and desires along that continuum. Further, an individual's place on that continuum can and does change throughout their lives. "Trans" is also accepted as an umbrella term and is becoming more popular, especially since there is a history of some tension between those identifying as transsexual versus transgendered (Koyama, 2001). In this article, trans and transgendered are used interchangeably, and both serve as umbrella terms describing a range of gender variant or gender non-conforming experiences, identities or expressions.

The Transgender Training Project of The New England AIDS Education and Training Center has been providing training on transgender-related issues to health-care providers in the New England region since 1999. The project has delivered 31 presentations to providers in the New England region, reaching over 600 people in workshop and conference settings. Additionally, the project has trained over 3,000 providers in other regions of the country.

The Transgender Training Project embarked on a study during the 2001-2002 grant year to interview providers of HIV-related care and advocacy on their knowledge and experience with working with transgendered people and to assess training needs to increase their effectiveness with transgendered clients. Below we will report on the study's findings.

METHODS

Participants

Participants were health-care providers involved in HIV-specific care who are affiliated with the New England AIDS Education and Training Center network and who have had some experience working with transgendered clients. Providers were recruited at the New England AIDS Education Center's annual meeting and through other contact information available through this agency. In some cases, the initial provider contacted referred another provider in their agency or practice who was then interviewed.

Thirteen interviews were conducted with clinicians (1 physician, 2 nurses, and 3 nurse practitioners), case managers (n = 4), and pharmacists (2 pharmacists and 1 pharmacy technician). Interviewees worked in Connecticut, Maine, Massachusetts, New Hampshire, and Vermont. Providers worked in urban, small city and rural settings. Worksites included community health centers, community-based clinics, community-based pharmacies, and HIV clinics in hospital settings.

Instruments

Interview questions were designed to discover information about:

1. knowledge and experience on transgender issues;
2. comfort with transgendered patients and provider-patient relationship;
3. challenges with provision of health care and referral;
4. HIV-related experience including Highly Active Anti-retroviral Therapy with HIV-positive transgendered patients, sexual history-taking, and risk reduction counseling;
5. agency-related barriers;
6. preferences for methods of training and learning.

The interview questions were pilot-tested with several providers as well as reviewed by a physician involved in transgender health care. In the pilot sessions, providers indicated that they and their colleagues would "feel uncomfortable being asked questions they didn't know the answers to." As a result, questions were reframed to be more open-ended and allow for more free-flowing responses. For example, instead of asking "How would you explain 'pre-op' and 'post op'?" the final question was "How does the medical community define 'Transgendered'?" Another example was to go from the specific "Are you familiar with the Harry Benjamin Standards of Care? What is your understanding of them?" to the more broad "What do you think are some challenges for providers in working with Transgendered people?" and "What are some specific things you would like to know more about?" (For a complete list of interview questions, please contact the author directly.)

Since many of the providers interviewed had no or little exposure to transgender medicine, and were not familiar with community definitions or language or the Harry Benjamin International Gender Dysphoria Association's Standards of Care (HBIGDA is the professional organization dedicated to treatment of transgender conditions), the final framing of the questions honored their areas of expertise while allowing them to identify gaps in training and information.

Procedure

Key informants were interviewed individually in their office setting. Interviews lasted from 45 minutes to an hour. Participants reviewed and signed an information and consent form and were given a choice of books on transgender health care for their personal libraries as a small token of appreciation for their contribution to the project. The interviews were audiotaped, transcribed and coded to determine themes.

RESULTS

Knowledge of Transgender Experience

All of the providers interviewed had had some experience with a transgendered patient or client, but many said that they were not necessarily familiar with terminology or distinctions within different communities. A number of providers explained understanding "transgender" to mean "medical intervention to move

from one gender to another gender" "as opposed to transvestites." Some explained "someone who is gender ambiguous but not having gone through a gender process." "Gender process" in this context referred to traditional gender reassignment, involving psychotherapy, hormone therapy and genital surgery.

But there was a range of thinking and an awareness that a broader view of gender nonconformity might not be common in the medical community. One experienced participant explained:

> Currently, the transgendered population is all over the map in terms of stages of reassignment they are going through. That's what I'm seeing. Have people intent on having complete gender reassignment and working towards that process. And have other patients who have no plans at all of ever going through that. And I have other patients who want to do certain components of it, may go through some. They might for instance, go through breast augmentation, but not genital surgery. But my colleagues are not with that definition. Providers with my mindset are few. . . . For the most part, the old way of looking at it, client says they are gender dysphoric, in the ways they can say it, usually psychologically, and then [providers] say how can we move this person along to full transition, from whatever, MTF or FTM. That is the standard.

Using a medical model to define a transgendered patient was more common among the clinical providers. One of the non-clinical providers offered an opposing definition that he thought was more common among his colleagues at an urban community-based clinic. His belief was that people were more likely to think of people who cross dress, who don't "pass," as transgendered.

> I know the definition of TG because I used to work with them. But I think that the people that I work with here? I think they define transgenders as cross dressers. If they are a man who dresses in women's clothing or a woman who dresses in men's clothing, they would consider

them transgendered. They call them drag queens. I think they mostly think about the male to female more than the female to male. I know that the term transgendered is more broader than that. The word "transgender" is an umbrella term and encompasses much more than that. Could be drag queens and drag kings, cross dressers, pre-ops, it can encompass a lot more than that. It is not necessarily the dress up piece but also the mental piece.

One important factor in providers' knowledge was the degree of their experience and exposure to transgendered people and the cultural norms that exist in different trans communities. When providers only have exposure in rare instances, they are not able to develop comfort and expertise.

I don't have repeated exposures to develop enough expertise. And that's one of the problems when you don't run into something a lot. I know that experience helps. I know where I was 15 years ago dealing with gay men.

Mental health providers might be very experienced around HIV, substance abuse, depression, but really don't have as much experience dealing with psychosocial challenges of someone who is transgendered.

The lack of experience influences a sense of discomfort on the part of providers, and this can then lead to unhelpful or even hostile treatment of the trans client. This can be based on lack of knowledge and discomfort.

When a person comes to [the provider's] site, there's no algorithm or context or training that they can rely on and I think what happens in that case is that people rely on what they do know, which may be neutral or may be negative, depending on their other life experiences.

Patients can also have extremely negative experiences, which might be due to lack of training and guidance, but also due to discrimination and bias against transgendered people.

One of the case managers described a hostile scene at a community health center.

The transgendered person was at central registration and the worker clearly laughed in their face. They just laughed at the person. And they kept demanding the person's birth name. And the person was identifying themselves by their transgender name. [The worker] laughed at the person and clearly made the person feel like they were not welcome. And that was in a "community" health center. They tried to get me involved in the "haha" joke, and when they saw that I didn't find it funny they were wondering what was wrong with me.

Providers Play a Role in Teaching Patients

Sometimes the provider has language or exposure that the client does not have. Even within the transgendered community, there is a range of awareness and of language. Not all self-describe as transgendered, some may have a bias against the word or simply not be aware of its meaning, and providers sometimes play a role in educating them and introducing them to the transgender community in a new way.

I've learned in working in this field to meet people where they're at. If they ID as male, and I clearly know them as female. I will ID them as male. But I'll let them know that there is another word for that, that it is transgender, I'll try to educate them around that. You know, "you may want to consider yourself to be transgendered."

Information is often needed to dispel myths and lack of information on the part of patients and their perceived risks. An example:

One patient, this was my most surprising situation. I had a FTM patient who had hypertrophy of the clitoris because of long-term use of testosterone and also he had bought a device that helped to enlarge the clitoris where it looked like a small penis, and he was in a relationship with a woman where he believed that he could impregnate her. And I had to go through–first of all my surprise, that you could think that–and then go and explain that the genitalia could change but that [capacity to impregnate] doesn't happen.

Dealing with Difference and Complexity

Working in the field of HIV, providers feel they are already situated in marginalized communities and more equipped to handle issues of difference and non-conformity in areas of sexuality, sexual expression and gender identity. HIV providers expressed that complexity of individuals' life and psychosocial challenges are built in to the relationship around issues of HIV prevention, risk assessment, and treatment.

> You expect, you're an HIV clinic, people in HIV work, expect to have folks of all sorts of stripes, quote "out of the norm." We deal with a wide variety of individuals marginalized in different ways. People come here who move in and out of society for many reasons.

There was a recognition that issues faced by transgendered people are many layered and that tools for cultural competency would be useful in training providers on how to work with this population.

> A challenge we have as providers is that we want to do targeted work, but someone who comes who is transgendered is not coming as one targeted thing. There are a lot of aspects, besides transgendered identity, that define that person's identity. You have to be able to understand that, part of it is to focus on the individual and part of it is to focus on the community and what its needs are.

> The problems that arise for transgendered people are multi-factorial. You have to look at them from all perspectives in order to provide comprehensive care.

Distinctions from Gay and Lesbian Services

Several of those interviewed self-identified as gay or lesbian or worked in gay, lesbian, bi-

sexual, and transgender (GLBT) agencies. Often, transgender lives and experiences are conflated with gay and lesbian experience. While there is overlap, for instance, effeminate men and masculine women have a strong presence in gay and lesbian communities, sexual orientation and gender identity are different things. Transgender people may identify as gay, lesbian, bisexual, heterosexual, pan-sexual, or a-sexual. Their sexual orientation may be based on their identity, not their anatomy. Thus, a male-to-female transwoman might identify as a straight woman in her relationships with men. A female-to-male transman might identify as a gay man if he is sexually attracted to or has sexual experiences with biologically male gay men.

It is not unusual for providers to miss the distinctions. For instance, one gay-identified provider said, "I think of people who are drag queens. I don't label them as transgendered. If they engage in sex with other men, I consider them as gay men."

Interviewees expressed reluctance on the part of their organizations to embrace transgendered people:

> People that work in this agency, they're all in a different place in terms of understanding. Some of us are like, we just have to do it [add transgender to our mission and focus]. But others resist. And I think the resistance is fear-based.

> We know that not including Transgender [in our agency name] we're doing a disservice. The B and the T are there, they're just not in our name. . . . To do it right, takes time. If you can't provide the services, you shouldn't add the letters. Need to know, what are the services we need to provide in order to add that to our name.

Building Trust for Effective Provider-Patient Relationships

Providers were uniformly well-intentioned and discussed how being able to focus on the client and build trust are necessary to create sufficient comfort for patients to open up, discuss and disclose risks, work through risk assessment and risk reduction plans, etc. Both medical providers and case managers who provide counseling said being accepting as a clinic and non-judgmental as a provider, letting clients know "anything you say in this exam room is fine," were key elements to building trust.

> How people get and receive care from a provider does depend on how comfortable that person feels with the provider. Many transgendered people have enough self work to do and enough self stuff going on that the last thing they want to do is train someone on their needs or the needs of the transgender community, so it becomes the provider's responsibility to have that information.

Obviously, there are limitations to the degree of trust, openness and success any counselor or provider can have with a client. Interviewees also recognized that the power imbalance inherent in provider/patient relationships plays a big role in the ultimate extent of that relationship, especially pertaining to such issues as gender non-conformity, drug use, sexual behavior and other activities that might be illegal or judged harshly by providers.

> Another thing we know is that people lie. And part of that is we don't want to expose ourselves to a person who may have a lot of power over our lives as a medical provider. If my experience in life is that you are going to withhold something [e.g., access to hormone therapy] from me, I'm going to lie. It's hard enough to tell these things to people who I know and trust. If I tell you, it could be a bad thing.

Understanding that there is a power relationship, but also wanting to build rapport, asking questions in an affirming way and not assuming to know what a client wants or needs were also seen as essential to effective interviewing.

> The point becomes how do we ask the question that's affirming, how do we value that person and get the information that we need.

One of the barriers is, not having an understanding of the person who is across from you, who is the patient. The second barrier that is related to that is treating them as if you know what their needs are. In a sense that you put them into a box. For instance, if they are biologically female and you're treating them as female, but they don't view themselves as female, that's going to create real barriers in the rapport that you have with that client and ultimately may turn them away from receiving services.

> Providers need to ask open-ended questions that are general in scope. So patients can answer as is appropriate to them. Can't ask "do you have anal sex" [and they believe it is vaginal sex] because you're not gonna get the right answer. I think that's part of the problem. As soon as one of those questions is asked, everything stops. You can't go any further with that person.

Lack of Time

While providers recognize key elements to successful interviewing, there are institutional barriers that stand in the way, regardless of a provider's personal intentions. Simply put, building trust takes time. Case managers and counselors have a little more time than the clinical providers, some can take as long as a client needs to get to the root of tough issues, but in general, providers have only a short period of time to meet with a client and must cover a range of medical concerns in that time.

> Physicians are really overwhelmed. Managed care has really changed things. The way we arrange medical care as a society, you're lucky if you get 10 or 15 minutes with a person. If you have 1 or 2 minutes, what can you really ask? We're saying "add this to what you're already doing, and we want you to do it well." It is a burden.

> Also, [building trust] takes a lot of talking. Here we have the luxury of half hour

visits. Cut that down to 15 minute visits, and if the person has medical problems, don't have time to do it. It's like if you're gonna open a door . . . If you're HIV positive, we have case managers to talk, but if HIV negative, we don't have that luxury.

Provider Discomfort

One of the largest single issues found in this study was discomfort with asking questions–"fear of saying the wrong thing"–and wanting skills on how to ask questions of a transgendered client. Providers expressed that "ignorance is a barrier. People [providers] are generally uncomfortable, just like society at large." Providers stated that they understood the importance of connecting with a client but expressed awkwardness and discomfort with the actual interview process.

> People don't know how to ask. Particularly if you don't know where someone is physically. How do you ask the questions? "Are you sexually active" is hard enough, to actually go into details is harder. Most people don't go further and ask "what kinds of activities do you do?" . . . How do you ask without seeming voyeuristic or prying.

As noted earlier, professionals working in HIV are typically more experienced asking difficult or awkward questions and working with clients who have experiences outside of the providers' comfort level. This experience is directly applicable to working with trans clients. There are commonalities in the skills that are developed in this work, and the ways in which providers feel frustrated with being unsuccessful in connecting with clients.

> Part of me thinks it isn't any different than asking any other awkward questions. Same basics of dealing with stuff you don't know about. Trying to set some comfort level. You just don't want to put people on the spot. You don't want to sound like you don't know what you're talking about. You don't want to make anybody uncomfortable. And frequently,

the easiest way to do that is to avoid everything. Or just be very ambiguous. These are ways of being really useless. You can avoid the awkwardness by saying "you always use condoms don't you?" Which isn't helpful.

Interviewing Skills and Limitations

Another issue related to discomfort had to do with a sense that providers would not necessarily know what to do next if a client disclosed their gender identity or gender issues and then would need services or assistance related to trans issues. Limitations in terms of time, skills, referral networks, and medical information all contribute to this concern. While interviewees stated that they might not know what to do with the information, they also said they wanted to know how to begin to ask the questions that would lead them there, so that the interaction could be useful, helpful and effective. There is a tension between wanting to help clients feel comfortable and being afraid of getting too much information and not knowing what to do with it.

> What do you do next if someone discloses? How do you ask the first question. If there's somebody you sense there's something going on around gender identity, how do you ask the first question?

> I think my biggest need is to get some skills on how to get conversations going. And then what to do with them. Balancing invasiveness with what I need to know to help this person figure out what they need.

> There's a limit in terms of how much I'm going to be able to go into a person's life. But how to make someone comfortable and ask questions that probably a lot of people haven't been asked before because we all sort of run around avoiding it. Then I start thinking, well, who are you to bring this up. But I would like to be able to do that.

Lack of Guidelines and Protocols for Hormone Therapy

How and why people access medical care is important to consider, particularly for populations that are resistant to or have had bad experiences with institutionalized care. For transgendered people, one primary motivation to access health is to obtain hormones. Hormones aid in masculinization and feminization for trans people, and play an essential part in their ability to live in their chosen gender role, both physically and emotionally. Providers acknowledged that they weren't very familiar with guidelines for prescribing and monitoring hormones, especially for clients who were also HIV positive.

Interviewees stated that the lack of standard guidelines for hormone therapy and other standard screening guidelines were a significant barrier in providing care. Additionally, lack of medical literature on effects of hormone therapy, particularly with other medications or conditions, made providers concerned about their ability to serve their clients and meet their health care needs.

> To effectively work with them, I think we don't offer the services that they necessarily want. If they come in for HIV counseling and testing, we can address that, if they come in for hepatitis vaccinations or STDs, we can address that, or women's clinic, we can address that. But if they come in for hormone therapy, we're not equipped to handle that. That is an area where we've been approached by people in the transgender community and we don't have the resources to provide that.

Hormones, Highly Active Anti-Retroviral Therapy (HAART) and HIV

Many comments were made about physicians' lack of knowledge about the effects and potential risks of hormone therapy and sex reassignment surgery for those living with HIV. There were two main areas of need and concern among the providers when it comes to the transgender-specific health needs of their HIV-positive patients. One was to recognize the importance of hormone therapy for transgendered people's general health and well-being, and the other was a frustration about the dearth of literature and expertise about combining hormone therapy and HIV medication regimens.

> What I have found is that a transgendered person is more likely, if they have to choose, which medication to let go of, hormones are first to hold on to. They would let go of HAART therapy or medications for other chronic diseases, but letting go of hormones is very difficult to negotiate. The gender reassignment seems to be the predominate drive. And a provider has to be sensitive to that, and respect that.

> Sometimes the person has to give up the hormones to take the meds and that's very traumatic for them. Because they are taking the hormones so they could be who they want to be. When they stop taking the hormones, their physical appearance changes, and I've seen them deal with that, it's very traumatic, and not a lot of people understand. [One client] died not long after they took her off the hormones. I just remember her being very depressed about it. She was very caught up on her looks. That was very important for her. When she knew she was dying, she requested a closed coffin, because she thought she wasn't beautiful.

In addition to a patient's emotional well-being being affected by hormone therapy, there are many specific questions about side effects, dosaging, long-term effects, co-infection with hepatitis and the like. Providers had many more questions than answers in this area and expressed frustration with lack of some of the most basic information.

> The whole issue of medications period. Since medications are processed in the liver. And when we're talking about a transgendered person, particularly MTF, dosages of hormones are very, very high, and then you're talking about combining that with HAART therapy, which is a

three drug regimen–all of which are processed in the liver . . .

We need to know: What are the medical implications, in terms of something as simple as what do you write on the referral, what are the medications people are using. Hormones and implications around interactions. I found out things theoretically, extrapolated. We know that some of the protease inhibitors will drop estrogen levels . . .

Particularly with HIV, we know that a lot of medications alter hormone levels. Oral contraceptive pills, thyroid medications, all those things need to be changed, how to actually manage somebody who is on hormone therapy who is also on protease inhibitors.

Lack of Expertise and Relevant Studies in the Literature

As in other evolving areas of medicine, expertise develops by providers who see a lot of patients and then somehow disseminate that information. But adequate, helpful professional consultation is also a need.

The person who takes care of a hundred people is gonna become the expert. What guidelines are they using? Who are the three or four experts in the U.S., get them to come up with basic guidelines.

It's very difficult to get information. I had my first [transgendered] patient, I didn't have a clue about hormones. Tried to reach people. Couldn't just get medical advice, "this is what you screen for, this is what you look for." A resource, like Hopkins has the AIDS Line, something like that, you could just click on for people taking care of transgendered patients, I think would be very helpful.

One provider who had extensive experience working with transgendered patients was very clear that the lack of literature and standards feels dangerous and irresponsible.

The literature that exists at this point is scanty at best. With transgender care, we don't know–Are we doing harm or not? There's no standard. I'm very concerned about long-term hormone use. Are we potentially doing harm? If we know that we can negotiate with our patients? I'm really into informed consent. This is part of our responsibility as providers.

Along with the lack of visible, well-known experts in the field, there is also a dearth of published literature that informs treatment decisions and informed consent.

Literature is not very broad compared to other areas of medicine where we have more than we can read at times. With transgender care and medicine, there are big gaps in information base. We don't really know the long-term effects of hormone therapy that we give, the doses that are given we have no idea as to the potential risk . . .

Because we don't have any long-term studies, don't know other potential risks or contraindications to use of high doses of hormones that we're not even fully aware of. We don't have the expertise in terms of endocrinology to assist us in this process.

Screening Guidelines

Another area of training need is the provision and dissemination of guidelines for providers in screening patients for transgender-specific care. The most widely used guidelines for gender reassignment are the Standards of Care for the Treatment of Gender Identity Disorders of the Harry Benjamin International Gender Dysphoria Association (available online at: *http://www.hbigda.org/socv6.html*), and these guidelines help providers establish some consistency in care and a potential consultation network. However, the guidelines focus on evaluation for hormone therapy and gender reassignment surgery, not on general screenings for primary health care maintenance. Providers offering maintenance and primary care have many questions:

If you have a standard set of screening guidelines for males and females, how do you figure out which ones you use for transgender patients? What do you do about osteoporosis, for example. How does that change?

The most concrete need is simply basic medical issues. Issues of screening, breast implants' potential risks, utilization of hormonal treatment, persistence of screening for prostrate cancer for male-to-females.

Providing Referrals

Both case managers and clinical providers act as advocates and mediators for their clients and in both cases, interviewees felt obligated to be able to provide quality, appropriate referrals. For transgendered clients, however, interviewees stated that they don't have a good professional network and often send clients to a provider without knowing if they can trust the reception or care that awaits the client.

An interviewee at a community-based GLBT clinic explained that he thought access to care in general for transgender patients is very limited:

I think that it is difficult because the transgendered people that we see here, when you talk to them about health care, they're not going anywhere. So that says to me that they're not going because they can't find providers who understand what the transgendered experience is all about. . . . As far as general health, we just send them off to people on our list, hoping that their needs get met.

Providers expressed struggles with what is normally a simple part of a referral–describing the patient and problem. But with trans clients, it gets complicated quickly. "What are the medical implications in terms of something as simple as what you write on a referral? How do you describe that person on a radiology request form when you refer for an MRI? I'll write down '43-year-old woman' and they put her under MRI machine and she's a pre-surgical transgender person."

Emergency Rooms and Hospitals

There was a sense that patients are better off within interviewees practice than outside of it. Stories of emergency room visits and hospital stays confirmed this impression.

An issue is: how to alert the emergency room. If they got admitted to the hospital, what amount of detail to explain to the nurses, how much detail did they want us to go into. One of them was initially very difficult for the nurses–they had no idea about how to deal with it, how to discuss it. It was a big issue about what room to put the person in. Had to negotiate it and when she was admitted, got put into a private room.

One patient who was in the hospital, once she got over her anger at how she was being treated, was pretty good about educating [the nursing staff]. We tried to have her always be on the same floor and with the same nurses, so that the nurses knew and became more sensitive around it.

Access to Substance Use Treatment Programs

One case manager related a particularly painful story about trying to access a drug treatment referral for a transgendered client. Substance use is well documented among transgendered people and being able to access appropriate drug treatment is a huge community need (Lombardi, 2000). In turn, providers need to know where to send someone for substance abuse treatment. The case manager described trying to help a trans woman who was getting out of prison and asked for his help in getting into a drug treatment program upon her release:

She knew she was getting out and if she spent any time on the streets she would pick up her habit again and I was trying to do something before she got out and I was unsuccessful. She wanted to go into a female residential treatment facility and the director said she wasn't a female. I was trying to explain she wasn't a threat to the other women. [The director] wasn't hearing it. The person had implants and had her testicles removed, but she had a penis. She started working the streets again and picked up her habit. Essentially I was pissed. I was really, really pissed. As far as I know, there's no transgender treatment center out there. If there is, I would love to know about it. There's not even one that is even sensitive to these issues. Putting an MTF in a male facility, that would be cruel.

Indeed, most substance use treatment programs are structured along binary gender lines, with patients often being placed according to their birth gender, obviously severely limiting their options regarding treatment.

Agency Issues

Above, under "Provider Discomfort," we addressed individual responsibilities of providers for building an effective relationship with their transgendered clients. But change must be system-wide as well. The climate of an agency, its policies, training, and location in the community all influence how transgendered people can access care.

The interviewees described significant issues that are institutionally based. Providers felt: (1) that agencies have a responsibility to be inclusive and to have policies in place for culturally competent treatment of trans people; (2) that making an agency welcoming should not be up to any one individual; (3) that individuals who want change within their agencies may not be empowered to create that change; (4) that there is transphobia and resistance among staff; and (5) that training and awareness must be across all levels of staff, including front desk staff.

Intake Forms, Frontline Staff and Insurance

Patients who come in to a clinic or agency have to interact with the receptionist, security staff and other people long before seeing a treatment provider. Regardless of the training or sensitivity level of the providers they will see later, that initial interaction is crucial to making a person feel welcome and safe. It is at the front

desk where issues of in-take forms, legal name versus preferred name, and insurance issues must be handled.

> I know working here the [sensitivity] training would even have to start at the front door. The frontline people that meet them at the door before I would even consider bringing a transgendered person in here and consider they could get care here.

> Do they train receptionists here? They should but they don't.

Some providers interviewed also felt that questions about past surgery or medications would capture a person's transgender status. It depends on how the questions are asked and how a provider reads and interprets the form.

> You first have to have in-take forms that offer T as one of the options. Or "other" and let them fill it in. I've actually had patients who leave it blank, and then I say "Why did you leave this blank." And that's another way to get at that information.

Insurance policies are often restrictive for transgendered people, with many insurance companies denying coverage for hormones or treatment related to gender reassignment. Providers in the study attested to these difficulties, starting at the level of listing gender and pronouns.

> Insurance forms [as they exist] are gender specific. A prescription is rejected if medication that is normally used for men or women is prescribed differently and they might reject it. It is absolutely a big potential problem.

> There's no deviation with insurance companies. We need another pronoun. I have a client who is intersexed. It's a slap in the face when genetically you aren't M or F.

Tension in Agencies About Trans Inclusion

Providers had stories of tension within their agencies over trans inclusion, including resistance, fear and outright discrimination. One interviewee who had worked for many years in a lesbian-oriented women's health clinic, an agency she had helped guide through many different changes, told this story:

> The issue came up on whether or not the organization would provide services to transgendered people. We struggled for many months. Many people did not want to do it. Since we were only seeing women, had to decide how we would draw the line. Said okay, we will see female-to-males pre-surgery and male-to-females post surgery. Surgery was the deciding factor. We had to do a lot of work, a lot of training, to come to the decision that "if you present yourself as a woman, then you are a woman and we will view you as a woman." So the whole discussion/argument/fight about pre- or post-surgery versus psychological identification. And we finally, though a lot of work, a lot of training, came to the decision that "if you present yourself as a woman, then you are a woman and we will view you as a woman." That it doesn't matter whether you have male genitalia or not. . . .

Another interviewee with a GLBT community health clinic acknowledged tension within the staff about actively pursuing and accepting transgendered clients.

> People that work in this agency, they're all in a different place in terms of understanding. Some of us are like, we just have to do it. But others resist. And I think the resistance is fear-based.

Training

An important domain of the interviews regarded methods for teaching and learning among health care professionals, and exploration of successes and failures on transgender topics specifically. This information could likely lead to more effective trans awareness programming, as well as help in planning for other methods of disseminating treatment information and research.

The following training needs and suggestions were identified in the interviews with the providers:

1. Staff at all levels should attend awareness training.
2. Have transgendered people as trainers.
3. Offer appropriate language to use in interviews, including role plays of specific interviewing skills.
4. Because of the potential challenge to get providers to attend a transgender-specific training, transgender issues may be better incorporated into broader trainings on diversity or other topics.
5. Utilize ways of training that are already institutionalized, such as journals, web pages, telephone "warm" lines, in-services, Grand Rounds, conferences.
6. Incorporate training in curriculum for medical students.

Sensitivity versus Knowledge

Among the providers who have had some exposure to transgender training, a distinction was made between gaining an understanding of the issues involved versus having the knowledge and skills to provide adequate care, treatment and counseling.

> When I think of the trainings I have done, they've been kind of similar, and not taken me farther, but it feels fresh each time that I do it. I feel like I'm sensitized, but not knowledgeable. I don't know how to take it to the next level.

> Clinicians don't even know that there are transgendered people. It's important to get them to take that seriously. After you did that, you could engage them in conversations about actual care.

Training Barriers

Providers cited difficulty in attracting people to trainings on transgender issues because of the many competing training needs that providers have, a lack of time, and sense that this issue isn't a priority. A suggestion was to incorporate trans issues into a training on a broader topic, such "Taking a Sexual History," or on prevention issues.

> If you did something solely on Transgenders, nobody would go. Because they have too much to do already. You have people who still need to get diabetes training, which they are seeing a lot of. Incorporate [trans information] into training that has to do with interviewing, or even around sexual history taking. Roll it into something they want to learn about. Make it part of half-day training on prevention.

Role Playing to Learn Interviewing Skills

Because providers were clear about needing actual interviewing skills, role plays were identified as an effective method for learning. Experiential learning, within a reasonable timeframe, is beneficial and effective for busy providers who need to learn a lot quickly. Interviewees expressed a desire for interview tools, such as a script with questions.

> Give them words to use, or the first questions, and you can use those and then come up with the words and style that works for you. I went to a lecture on sexual history taking and I was like, I wouldn't say it that way, but I've been doing this for a long time. If I hadn't then it is good to have the actual words to use. Tell me just three sentences as intro sentences, and I'll try those.

> I don't have repeated exposures to develop enough of an expertise. And that's one of the problems when you don't run into something a lot. But if there were something, probably role playing is the way to do it, watching someone and then doing it. Video, vignette, actually hear words and get to hear how they sound to you. Then maybe you can use those words for the first time.

Importance of Transgendered People as Trainers

Interviewees felt very strongly that transgendered people needed to be involved in the design and delivery of trainings for providers. They stated that hearing personal experiences

and being able to see the provider-patient relationships through the transgendered person's eyes would have a strong impact on the quality of care. Additionally, it was noted that the trans person doing the training would need to have training skills and come across as empowered, charismatic and knowledgeable.

> Inviting a transgendered person here. Someone who is very comfortable in their skin. And who is comfortable talking about transgendered issues. Who possibly even works in the field. Who knows all the idiotic and stupid questions that people probably would ask, who would subject themselves to having case managers and health educators ask them any kind of questions . . . Sort of open themselves up to questions.

> You have to have members of the population present to talk about their own experiences to get the full spectrum of what gender reassignment means. Again, the multidisciplinary approach is really essential.

> It would be helpful for someone to guide us through what it feels like to be on the other end of the exam table. To help us think about how we talk to our patients–having someone who is transgendered come and talk to us.

One provider stated "I've been extensively trained by my patients. They teach me things all the time." On the other hand, providers recognized that it can be a burden for patients to educate their health care providers and that providers may have to go elsewhere to seek out information about transgendered people and their lives. Further, it was recognized that one patient cannot educate a provider about all trans people.

> I also could learn a lot by sitting down with a patient. Although I think there are a lot of people who are sick of having to educate their providers, the same way people with HIV are sick of having to teach their providers this and that. So I don't know specifically about transgendered people, but I think people expect more of their providers than having to educate them, even though a lot of people take that role on pretty nicely.

DISCUSSION

Transgendered people are emerging as a visible group that is at high risk for HIV, and clearly there are many information and training needs for HIV providers who are, (or will be), working with members of this population. The lack of studies and difficulty accessing information will continue to impact how well providers can offer care. At the same time, as providers in this study noted, their comfort level will naturally improve as they grapple with increased experience and exposure to transgendered patients. This small study is a beginning step in identifying the many areas in which research, training and information are needed, and identifies some effective ways to deliver that information.

In summary, we found that providers had:

1. Desire to treat transgendered patients respectfully, but admitted discomfort and lack of tools for specific interviewing/ assessments.
2. Experience with a range of transgendered patients, but lacked information on distinctions among transgendered experiences.
3. Restrictions based on time constraints that create an overarching barrier in building trusting relationships with clients, and trusting relationships are integral to quality care.
4. Concern and frustration with lack of information, studies and research.
5. Concern and frustration with lack of treatment guidelines, (or ability to access them), referral contacts and ways to advocate for transgender clients.
6. Belief that training by transgendered people themselves was an essential teaching element.

Limitations

This was a small qualitative study, based on only 13 interviews. The providers interviewed here all volunteered their time and were interviewed face-to-face, indicating their commitment and interest to this issue. They are best perceived as representative of providers who work in HIV and want to improve their capacity for providing compassionate care to this marginalized group. While transgendered people have identified bias and discrimination as barriers to care, in this group, the greatest barriers were lack of experience and access to information. Their honest assessment of barriers and limitations provide useful evidence for the development of training curricula and strategies. Further data gathering from this group will continue to justify and inform training programs.

Research Is Needed

The need for research is abundantly clear. Any medical database search will turn up amazingly little on transgendered people and health care, even less on the effects of HIV or HIV medications with transgendered patients. Providers acknowledged that this lack of information–on dosages, risks, complications, drug interactions and co-morbidities–prevent them from being able to partner with their patients on decision-making and informed consent.

Pharmaceutical companies also have an obligation to include transgendered people in studies. As remarkable as it may seem, the use of hormone therapy for gender reassignment is off-label. No studies have been conducted by pharmaceutical companies on use of hormones in gender transition, again, leaving providers and patients virtually in the dark about long-term concerns and reinforcing the invisibility and disregard of transgendered lives in traditional areas of medicine.

There are a number of barriers related to this lack of research. Lack of funding, and indifference to the topic by researchers are among them. But where transgendered lives are considered, there is still a great deal of misunderstanding. For example, the federal Centers for Disease Control, which controls HIV-prevention funding and thus the direction of most prevention efforts, categorizes all transgendered people in the risk category of men who have sex with men, or MSM. This fails to recognize that many male-to-female transgendered people who have male sex partners consider themselves to be women in heterosexual relationships. Their partners also see the relationship as heterosexual. Categorizing these men and women as MSM fails to recognize the identity and experience of the population and cannot result in useful risk assessment or the development of effective programs (Xavier, 2000; Kenagy, 2002; Kammerer, 1996 and Clements-Nolle, 1999).

This example also shows a lack of distinction between gender identity and sexual orientation. It is common for community agencies and health centers who have historically served gays and lesbians to now use the initials "GLBT," or gay, lesbian, bisexual and transgendered, to define their target population. People who identify as transgendered may, in fact, identify as straight, gay, bisexual or even something else to categorize their sexual orientation. The letters "GLBT" are often used to express inclusion of sexual and gender minorities within the same movement or organizational mission. The differences are important for agencies and providers to recognize, and it is also important to recognize that some transgender people have specific negative experiences within the gay and lesbian communities (Clements-Nolle, 1999 and McGowan, 1999). Yet, there remains an urge to conflate sexual orientation, particularly homosexuality, with transgender identity.

In 1999, the American Public Health Association issued a policy resolution addressing this tendency. "The Need for Acknowledging Transgendered Individuals within Research and Clinical Practice" concluded "that transgendered individuals are not receiving adequate health care, information or inclusion within research studies because of discrimination by and/or lack of training of health care providers and researchers, urges the National Institutes of Health and the Centers for Disease Control (as well as individual researchers and health care workers) to categorize MTF and FTM transgendered individuals as such and not conflate them with gay men or lesbians (unless appropriate to an individual's sexual orientation in their preferred gender) as well as acknowledging the variation that exists among transgendered individuals" (Lombardi, 1999).

Recognizing the variation among transgendered people can also lead to broader research areas. For instance female-to-male transgendered people, or trans men, are ignored altogether in the CDC categorizations, yet this is a subpopulation becoming more widely visible. Some data gathering is starting to ask questions about FTM lives and sexual risk behaviors, but it is largely an ignored category, leaving HIV-positive FTMs, or FTMs with HIV-positive partners with little information on treatment or secondary prevention.

With such a longstanding history of tension from and mistrust of the medical system, it is also a challenge to recruit transgendered people as participants in studies. Having transgendered people involved in designing research projects can help build trust and create a climate where participants of a minority group are tapped and acknowledged for their contributions to developing areas of health care. Building this culture of partnership between researchers, providers and patients will result in studies that will begin to fill the gaps in information and enlighten standards and options for care.

Once the research is done, it needs to be disseminated quickly. In an area with such little research and information, studies should be released widely using various methods of distribution, including web sites such as the AIDS Education and Training Center's National Resource Center and the National HIV/AIDS Clinician Consultation Center.

Treatment Protocols and Standards of Care

The Harry Benjamin International Gender Dysphoria Association, or HBIGDA, Standards of Care are the best known guidelines, but they are geared towards assessing eligibility and readiness for hormone therapy and sex reassignment surgery and are not guidelines for ongoing medical care. The HBIGDA is an international professional association for a range of providers (surgeons, psychologists, endocrinologists, sociologists, etc.) and has an active and committed membership that includes many transgendered people.

The "Benjamin Standards," or SOC, as they are known, have been criticized for limiting patient's autonomy and creating a "gatekeeper" relationship whereby patients need a provider's, usually a psychotherapist, approval for hormones. "The real lives of transgendered people might be more complex or divergent from the guidelines and patients may not feel they can be honest with their physicians if termination of hormonal therapy is a possibility" (Karasic, 2000). However, this criticism seems to have been directly addressed with the development of more recent versions of the SOC that allow for much more flexibility (Standards of Care for Gender Identity Disorders, Sixth Version). It might be most useful to see the SOC as a companion to other documents that give screening and treatment guidance to physicians.

One of these documents is "Medical Care of Transgendered Patients" (Oriel, 2000), which is founded in the Benjamin Standards and also offers clinical guidelines for practitioners. "Transsexual patients often have difficulty finding care because many physicians are not comfortable prescribing appropriate hormone regimens. Management of hormones for transsexual patients is not difficult and these medications are safer than many therapies routinely prescribed by the primary care physicians. . . . This review is intended to teach primary care providers how to initiate and maintain hormone regimens for transsexual patients and describe medical issues unique to transsexual patients."

Several clinics are establishing their own protocols. Guidelines established by the Tom Waddell Health Center in San Francisco (Protocols for Hormonal Reassignment of Gender from the Tom Waddell Health Center, 2001) are available on the Web and are being used by clinics working with low-income, high-risk transgendered patients who seek access to hormone therapy. The Michael Callen-Audre Lorde Community Health Center in New York City (Callen-Lorde Protocols for the Provision of Hormone Therapy, 2001) has developed extremely detailed protocols for providers, outlining specific instructions for numerous visits with different categories of patients, samples of consent forms, and tables of contraindications and side effects. These guidelines can help increase the numbers of providers able to confidently treat transgendered patients and increase the number of clinics willing to provide hormone therapy as part of primary care with patients. Both agencies allow other clinics access to their documents to create their own protocols.

Providing hormones as part of primary care attracts transgendered patients and also allows them to have access to HIV prevention or treatment information. Providing this access directly addresses HIV risk by eliminating the alternative means of accessing hormones–using street market hormones, sharing needles and vials, and having no ongoing monitoring regarding dosaging, complications or risks. A successful program in New York entitled "The HIV Hormone Bridge" (Grimaldi et al., 1996, 1998) drew impoverished HIV-positive sex workers to HIV care by offering hormone therapy as part of a broader treatment contract and community program. The program was successful in creating community for participants through support groups and building self-esteem; and in helping transgender patients develop trust for their providers, dramatically decreasing risk-taking activities such as use of street hormones and increasing medical compliance and receptivity to HIV medication.

Access to sex reassignment surgery, or SRS, is also an important need for many transgendered people, and the presence of HIV complicates this surgery, as it does all major surgeries. Some research and guidelines for SRS and HIV-positive patients have been developed, including two appearing in the *International Journal of Transgenderism* (Kirk, S., 2001, Wilson, N. A., 2001).

Final Recommendations

The findings from this study fall under three main areas. All three areas need to be addressed in providing training for providers, including skills related to relational and systems issues, encouraging advocacy and policy change, and facilitating linkages to informational resources. The three areas are:

1. *relational*, relationship between provider and patient; provider and transgender community; provider and his or her referral network;
2. *informational*, related to research, scientific literature, guidelines and expertise available for review and consultation; and
3. *systems*, how institutions (agencies, insurance companies, hospitals, and society at large) incorporate policy and procedure and attitudes related to transgendered patients.

Based on the findings of this study, recommendations in the three areas are:

Relational

- Training should be provided by transgendered people.

- Trainings must be easily accessible with concrete take-home messages given in a short period of time.
- Awareness training should be provided for all levels of staff.
- Skills for increasing comfort and competence in interviewing, especially sexual history taking and risk assessment should be stressed.
- Transgender awareness should be included in curriculum of broader topics, such as sexual history taking or prevention.
- Transgender Health subcommittees should be established in HIV/AIDS health care associations such as the Association of Nurses in AIDS Care.

Informational

- Research and dissemination of findings on long-term health risks of hormone therapy and sex reassignment surgery.
- Research and dissemination of findings on hormone treatment for HIV-positive transgendered people.
- Establishment of transgender categories in HIV risk assessment and transmission categories in all data collection efforts.
- Establishment and dissemination of guidelines for medical care for transgendered people and for transgendered people living with HIV.
- Availability of Continuing Medical Education on Transgender Health issues.
- Utilization of information systems such as the AIDS Education and Training Center's National Resource Center's website for central location of information for providers.

Systems

- Utilize existing training mechanisms–in-services, quarterly meetings, Grand Rounds, professional conferences–to present information.
- Incorporate transgender health information as part of regular curriculum in professional schools (medical school, nursing school, social work school, etc.).
- Advocate for and create changes in intake forms to include expanded gender choices and options for chosen versus legal name.

- Have agency policies and guidelines in place, including disciplinary procedures for mistreatment of transgendered clients.
- Create resources such as sample policy and procedures, forms, checklists and planning strategies for agencies wanting to become trans inclusive.
- Normalization of transgendered people in institutional settings, and information on appropriate care for transgendered patients in hospitals, emergency rooms, insurance companies, etc.
- Work to destigmatize gender non-conformity and gender variance to increase safety for transgendered people to disclose their status.

CONCLUSION

This study showed enormous gaps in knowledge, literature, professional expertise and skills around addressing the needs of transgendered patients living with or at risk for HIV. But this study also showed a sincere concern and desire on the part of providers to serve trans clients effectively. The challenge in designing and delivering trainings will be to strike a balance between providers' many demands for their time, institutional limitations related to policy and staff turnover, and the evolving visibility of trans communities demanding access to quality care.

REFERENCES

Bockting, W.O., Robinson, B.E., Rosser, B.R. Transgender HIV prevention: A qualitative needs assessment. *AIDS Care*, (1998), *10*:505-525.

Bockting, W. and Kirk, S., editors, *Transgender and HIV: Risks, prevention and care*. Binghamton, NY: The Haworth Press, Inc. (2001) Originally published as a special issue of *International Journal of Transgenderism 3.1+2*. Available online at *http://www.symposion/ijt*.

Bockting, W. *Transgender HIV prevention: A Minnesota response to a global health concern*, Collection of papers, W. O. Bockting, Minneapolis, Minnesota (1998).

Callen-Lorde Protocols for the Provision of Hormone Therapy, (2001). For information or to order a copy of the protocols, contact Wendy Stark, Associate Executive Director, Michael Callen-Audre Lorde Community Health Center, 212-271-7277.

Clements-Nolle, K., Marx, R., Guzman, R., & Katz, M. (2001, June). HIV prevalence, risk behaviors, health care use, and mental health status of transgender persons: Implications for public health intervention. *American Journal of Public Health, 91(6)*, 915-921.

Clements, K., Wilkinson, W., Kitano, K., & Marx, R. (1999). HIV prevention and health service needs of the transgender community in San Francisco. *International Journal of Trangenderism 3.1+2. http://www.symposion/ijt/hiv_risk/clements.htm.*

Grimaldi, J., Jacobs, J. (1998). The HIV Hormone Bridge: Connecting impoverished HIV+ transsexual sex workers to HIV medical care. Abstract presented at International Conference on AIDS Conference, 1998.

Grimaldi, J.M., Jacobs, J. (1996). HIV/AIDS transgender support group: Improving care delivery and creating community. Abstract presented at Int Conf AIDS, 1996 Jul 7-12; 11(1):421.

Dean, L., Meyer, I., Robinson, K., Sell, R., Sember, R., Silenzio, V., Bowen, D., Bradford, J., Rothblum, E., Scout, D., White, J., Dunn, P., Lawrence, A., Wolfe, D., Xavier, J. (2000). Lesbian, Gay, Bisexual, and Transgender Health: Findings and Concerns. *Journal of the Gay and Lesbian Medical Association 4(3)*: 105-151. *http://www.glma.org/pub/jglma/vol4/3/index.html.*

Elifson, K.W., Boles, J., Posey, E. et al. Male transvestite prostitutes and HIV risk. *American Journal of Public Health (1993)*, 83:260-262.

Feinberg, L. (2001). Trans health crisis: For us it's life or death. *American Journal of Public Health*. 2001; 91:897-900.

Gay and Lesbian Medical Association and LGBT health experts (2001, April). *Companion Document for Lesbian, Gay, Bisexual, and Transgender (LGBT) Health*. San Francisco: Gay and Lesbian Medical Association. *http://www.glma.org/policy/hp2010/index.html.*

GLBT Health Access Project, JSI Research & Training Institute, Inc. (2000). *Access to Health Care for Transgendered Persons in Greater Boston*. Boston: JSI Research & Training Institute, Inc.

GLBT Health Access Project (2001), *Community Standards of Practice for Provision of Quality Health Care Services for Gay, Lesbian, Bisexual and Transgendered Clients*, JRI Health, Boston, MA, *www.glbthealth.org.*

Harry Benjamin International Gender Dysphoria Association (February 20, 2001). *Standards of Care for Gender Identity Disorders, Sixth Version. http://www.hbigda.org/socv6.html.*

Health Law Standards of Care for Transsexualism. Second International Conference on Transgender Law and Employment Policy (1993). Available online at *http://www.altsex.org/transgender/healthlaw.html.*

Israel, G. & Tarver, D. (1997). *Transgender care: Recommended guidelines, practical information, and personal accounts*. Philadelphia: Temple University Press.

Kammerer, C.A., Hope Mason, T., Conners, M.M., Transgenders and HIV risks: Needs assessment. Prepared by the Massachusetts Department of Public Health, HIV/AIDS Bureau. August 1995. Reprinted in *Transgender and HIV: Risks, prevention and care*, ed. by W.O. Bockting and S. Kirk, Chapter 2, The Haworth Press, Inc., 2001.

Kammerer, N., Mason, T., & Connors, M. (1999). Transgender health and social service needs in the context of HIV risk. *International Journal of Trangenderism 3.1+2. http://www.symposion.com/ijt/hiv_risk/kammerer. htm.* Reprinted in *Transgender and HIV: Risks, prevention and care*, ed. by W.O. Bockting and S. Kirk, Chapter 3, The Haworth Press, Inc., 2001.

Karasic, D.H. (2000). Progress in Health Care for Transgendered People, Editorial, *Journal of the Gay and Lesbian Medical Association, 4(4)* 157-158.

Keatley, J. and Clements-Nolle, K. (2001). Factsheet: What are the Prevention Needs of Male-to-Female Transgender Persons? University of California, San Francisco, Center for AIDS Prevention Studies.

Kenagy, G.P. (2002). HIV among transgendered people, *AIDS Care, 14(1)* 127-134.

Kirk, S. (2001). Guidelines for Selecting HIV-Positive Patients for Genital Reconstructive Surgery, *Transgender and HIV: Risks, prevention and care*. Binghamton, NY: The Haworth Press, Inc. (2001). Originally published in *International Journal of Transgenderism 3.1+2*. Available online at *http://www.symposion/ijt.*

Lombardi, E. (2000, March). APHA Policy Statement, Resolution 9933: The need for acknowledging transgendered individuals within research and clinical practice, *American Journal of Public Health, 90(3)* 482-484.

Lombardi, E., van Servellen, G. (2000). Building culturally sensitive substance use prevention and treatment programs for transgendered populations, *Journal of Substance Abuse Treatment (19)* 2000. 291-296.

Lombardi, E. (2001, June). Enhancing transgender health care. *American Journal of Public Health, 91(6)*, 869-972.

Medical and Behavioral Health Guidelines for Transgendered Clients, Sydney Borum Jr. Health Center, Boston, MA.

McGowan, C. K. (1999). *Transgender Needs Assessment*. NY: The Prevention Planning Unit of the New York City Department of Health.

Namaste, V. K. (1999). HIV/AIDS and female to male transsexuals and transvestites: Results from a needs assessment in Quebec. *International Journal of Transgenderism 3.1+2. http://www.symposion.com/ijt/hiv_risk/namaste.htm.*

Nemoto, T., Luke, D., Mamo, L., Ching, A., & Patria, J. (1999). HIV risk behaviors among male-to-female transgenders in comparison with homosexual or bisexual males and heterosexual females. *AIDS Care, (11)*, 297-312.

Oriel, K. A. (2000). Medical care of transsexual patients. *Journal of the Gay and Lesbian Medical Association 4(4)*: 185-193.

Post, P. (2002). Crossing to Safety: Transgender Health and Homelessness, *Healing Hands: A publication of the Health Care for the Homeless Clinician's Network, 6(4),* June 2002.

Protocols for Hormonal Reassignment of Gender from the Tom Waddell Health Center, 2001, http://hivinsite.ucsf.edu/InSite.jsp?doc=2098.3d5a.

Rachlin, K. (2002). FTM 101: Dispelling myths about the invisible and the impossible, in *Female to Male Transexuals, The Phallus Palace,* edited by Dean Kotula, Los Angeles: Alyson Publications.

Sandoval, C. (1995). Transgendered Persons in California, Focus Groups Findings, Polaris Research and Development Inc. Available online at *http://hivinsite.ucsf.edu/InSite.jsp?doc=2098.3a57.*

St. Claire, R. (2001). Culturally-Sensitive Transgender Health Care, Transgender Soul–The Psychology of Transgender Issues. *http://www.transgenderesoul.com.*

Substance Abuse and Mental Health Services Administration. (2001). A provider's introduction to substance abuse treatment for lesbian, gay, bisexual and transgender individuals. Rockville, MD: Substance Abuse and Mental Health Services Administration, Center for Substance Abuse Treatment.

Wilkerson, G. (aka Williams, B.). (2001). What We Don't Know: The Unaddressed Health Concerns of the Transgendered, *Trans-Health.com (1)1. http://www.trans-health.com/Iss1Vol1?dont_know.htm.*

Wilson, N. A. (2001). Sex Reassignment Surgery in HIV-Positive Individuals, *Transgender and HIV: Risks, prevention and care.* Binghamton, NY: The Haworth Press, Inc. (2001). Originally published in *International Journal of Trangenderism 3.1+2.* Available online at *http://www.symposion/ijt.*

Xavier, J., & Simmons, R. (2000). *The Washington transgender needs assessment survey,* Washington, DC: The Administration for HIV and AIDS of the District of Columbia Government. See also: Xavier, J., & Simmons, R. (2000). *The executive summary of the Washington Transgender needs assessment survey. http://www.gender.org/vaults/wtnas.html.*

Gender as an Obstacle in HIV/AIDS Prevention: Considerations for the Development of HIV/AIDS Prevention Efforts for Male-to-Female Transgenders

Sheilla Rodríguez-Madera, PhD
José Toro-Alfonso, PhD

SUMMARY. Social discourses regarding gender are responsible for molding people's cognitions, perceptions, behaviors, and interactions with others. Approaching and understanding gender socialization is an important strategy that must be included in the development of HIV/AIDS prevention intervention efforts targeting male-to-female (MTF) transgender people.

This paper represents an effort to identify the influence of gender construction among a group of MTF transgenders in Puerto Rico. Using combined methodology, authors examined results from a questionnaire and in-depth interviews with a convenience sample of MTF transgenders living in the San Juan metropolitan area.

Quantitative analysis demonstrated that this sample is composed of young, unemployed, and undereducated population. Many participated in the sex industry. Participants reported need for basic health and social services and alienation from social networks. Qualitative analysis confirmed their traditional social construction of the "feminine." Their discourse underlines their need to reinforce their identity by the construction of a female self which undermines their possibilities for negotiating safer sex, as happens to most females in Latino societies.

Social vulnerability, institutional exclusion, and gender construction issues are obstacles for the HIV prevention efforts among these communities. *[Article copies available for a fee from The Haworth Document Delivery Service: 1-800-HAWORTH. E-mail address: <docdelivery@haworthpress. com> Website: <http://www.HaworthPress.com> © 2005 by The Haworth Press, Inc. All rights reserved.]*

KEYWORDS. Sex work, prostitution, HIV/AIDS, Latino, transgender, gender ideology

INTRODUCTION

The transgender label encompasses all individuals who defy traditional gender roles. This variety of gender identities include drag queens, androgynous, transvestites, transformers, intersexuals, transsexuals, and even particular fashion statements (American Educational Gender

Sheilla Rodríguez-Madera, PhD, and José Toro-Alfonso, PhD, are both affiliated with the University Center for Psychological Research and Services, Department of Psychology, University of Puerto Rico, San Juan, PR.

Address correspondence to: Sheilla Rodríguez-Madera, PhD, CUSEP/UPR, P.O. Box 23174, San Juan, PR 00931-3174 (E-mail: sheillalrm@hotmail.com).

[Haworth co-indexing entry note]: "Gender as an Obstacle in HIV/AIDS Prevention: Considerations for the Development of HIV/AIDS Prevention Efforts for Male-to-Female Transgenders." Rodríguez-Madera, Sheilla, and José Toro-Alfonso. Co-published simultaneously in *International Journal of Transgenderism* (The Haworth Medical Press, an imprint of The Haworth Press, Inc.) Vol. 8, No. 2/3, 2005, pp. 113-122; and: *Transgender Health and HIV Prevention: Needs Assessment Studies from Transgender Communities Across the United States* (ed: Walter Bockting, and Eric Avery) The Haworth Medical Press, an imprint of The Haworth Press, Inc., 2005, pp. 113-122. Single or multiple copies of this article are available for a fee from The Haworth Document Delivery Service [1-800-HAWORTH, 9:00 a.m. - 5:00 p.m. (EST). E-mail address: docdelivery@haworthpress.com].

Available online at http://www.haworthpress.com/web/IJT
doi:10.1300/J485v08n02_10

Services, 2001; Bockting, Robinson, & Rosser, 1998; Lunievicz, 1996). Still, it is important to emphasize that this concept does not completely explain the complexity and heterogeneity of the gender spectrum due to the multiple possibilities that exist in sexualities and gender identifications.

Due in part to prejudice, transgenders constitute an invisible and forgotten group in general, and particularly among Latino communities. This situation has serious health implications given the fact that studies have identified a great number of transgenders who are infected with HIV/AIDS or who engage in high risk sexual behaviors (Clements-Nolle, Marx, Guzman, & Katz, 2001; Rodríguez-Madera & Toro-Alfonso, 2000; Sykes, 1999). The number of transgenders infected with HIV is increasing, as evidenced by the 3% to 8% augment in new reported cases per year in the United States (Center for AIDS Prevention Studies, 2001). Until recently, the impact of the HIV/AIDS epidemic on the transgender community has been largely ignored (Bockting & Kirk, 2001) due to the fact that epidemiologically, they are included within the statistics of men who have sex with men. This is clearly another testament to their social invisibility.

It is important to work towards the legitimization of transgender people by understanding the ways in which they define, construct, and manifest their gender identities and sexualities, the factors that make them socially vulnerable, and the attitudes and beliefs that place them at risk for HIV/AIDS infection.

Motivated by this challenge, we decided to focus on one of the most important factors that are related to HIV risk among transgenders: gender socialization. Gender is a social construction that influences many dimensions of human beings. Moreover, social discourses regarding gender are responsible for molding people's cognitions, perceptions, behaviors, and interactions with others. Approaching and understanding gender socialization is an extremely important strategy that must be included in the development of HIV/AIDS prevention efforts among male-to-female (MTF) transgenders.

In this study with 50 MTF Puerto Rican transgenders, we collected data using a mixed method approach (Tashakkori & Teddlie, 1998)

in order to identify some of the social discourses about the "feminine" that tend to render MTFs vulnerable to HIV infection. The study results support our thesis that MTF transgenders face disadvantages similar to those experienced by women due to the way the feminine gender is constructed in patriarchal societies, in addition to the other socio-structural barriers that transgenders find in their daily lives. These obstacles are mainly due to the fact that modern western society identifies the transgender identities as transgressive, in that it challenges normative discourses imposed by the gender binomial.

The Social Construction of Gender and Its Implication for the HIV Epidemic

Our society promotes the development and perpetuation of dichotomous and exclusive categories (Wallach-Scott, 1999). Far from understanding that elasticity and fluidity characterize the development and transformation of identities, these are presented as rigid and static. Gender is one of the most important categories in society. Through it, the world is divided between the "feminine" and the "masculine." Indeed, gender identity is an organizing principle of unequal power relationships (Vance, 1999) which responds to the particular needs of social groups that use it as a means of social control. Traditionally, from the moment of birth a person's gender is determined by his/her sexual anatomy. Afterwards, people construct their gender identity in agreement with social discourses that establish what is appropriate for each gender (Wallach-Scott, 1999). Even sexual anatomy has been assumed as destiny. Gender and sexuality are expressions based on sexual differentiation which organized perception and interpretation (Nakano-Glenn, 1999). The sexed human subject can not be accounted for simply by categorizing people as male or female based on anatomical phenomena; this process is more complex (Collazo-Valentín, 1999).

Together, the State and society produce social discourses regarding gender and perpetuate them through social institutions like science, family, and religion. In the flowchart presented in Figure 1, we can see that these discourses influence a person's perception of his/

FIGURE 1. Social Discourses Flowchart

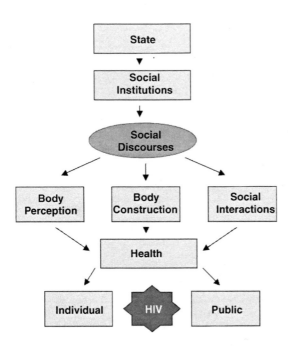

herself and the way he/she interacts with other people. This is relevant to the issue of HIV infection since these social discourses not only "construct" an individual with a weak perception of his/her abilities to negotiate safer sex practices, but they also have a great impact on the individual's social interactions. That is why in issues presented by the HIV/AIDS pandemic, gender socialization extends beyond the individual level, to the broader implications of public health (Varas Díaz & Toro-Alfonso, 2001).

Traditionally, in patriarchal societies, the male gender has been assumed to be powerful, controlling of the feminine, rational, strong, and sexually assertive (Butler, 1993). In direct contrast, the feminine gender has been characterized as weak, emotional, sensitive, dependent, and passive. Research has documented that, due to this dichotomous gender socialization, women face serious difficulties while engaging in negotiation of safer sexual practices (Ortiz-Torres, Serrano-García, & Torres-Burgos, 2000). This has direct implications on the dynamics of intimate sexual relations in the context of couples. This phenomenon, in part, could explain why women constitute the sec-

ond highest risk group for HIV infection in Puerto Rico (PASET, 2001).

Although feminist struggles have transformed widely held conceptions regarding the feminine gender, most MTF transgenders reproduce traditional patriarchal gender roles (Flecha Cruz, 2000; Kammerer, Mason, Connors, & Durkee, 2001). This is alarming, since the adoption of these roles presents the same disadvantages and difficulties that women face to engage in safer sexual practices. Understanding this issue is of vital importance, as studies have identified that sexual intercourse without a condom is one of the factors that places MTF transgenders at risk of HIV infection (Namaste, 2000; Rodríguez-Madera & Toro-Alfonso, 2000; Sykes, 1999). This is one of the reasons that gender construction must be addressed in preventive interventions with transgenders.

Other important issues related to condom use have to be considered as well. One such issue is that many transgenders work in the sex industry and there are clients who pay more money to have sexual intercourse without a condom. Considering that sex industry workers often have a precarious financial status it may be tempting to engage in such practices (Toro-Alfonso, 1995). In addition, Kammerer, Mason, Connors, and Durkee (2001) have identified the "conviction versus confusion debate," which entails two important perspectives. First, it might be difficult for clients to assume their responsibility about condom use when there is a denial of the other's penis as their object of desire. In other words, they are confused about their sexual identities and sexual orientation so they will not ask to use condoms because it can intensify their confusion. Second, the transgender will not suggest condom use in order to strengthen her gender identity. Using a condom would be a contradiction to their feminine imaginary. Not addressing the existence of their penis gives them a conviction of their gender. Both perspectives are important to explore and consider in preventive intervention designs.

It is obvious that in order to understand the transgender phenomenon we must account for factors that influence the development of gender identities. Thus, those who embody a paradigmatic shift regarding gender and question the established social order pay deeply. The consequences are evidenced in their physical, psychological, social and sexual functioning (Ettner, 1999). Due to the fact that gender construction issues are so complex and relative from one culture to another, it is important to explore exactly how the process of becoming a "woman with a penis" can make transgenders vulnerable to HIV infection in particular contexts.

HIV/AIDS and Transgenders in Puerto Rico: An Overview

The lives of the transgender people in the Puerto Rican context are characterized by experiences of oppression and discrimination. In a patriarchal society in which *machismo* rules, MTF transgenders represent a challenge to traditional masculinity due to their renouncing of the male position of social power. That is why MTF transgenders are more frequently targets of hate crimes and prejudice than are female-to-male transgenders.

The discrimination toward transgenders encompasses multiple levels. As in many other countries, these individuals are victims of: (1) rejection by their families, the community in general, and the gay community in particular, (2) lack of access to health services, (3) poverty, (4) substance use and abuse, and (5) physical and emotional abuse, among others (Bockting, Rosser, & Scheltema, 1999; Bockting, Robinson, & Rosser, 1998; Califia, 1999; Lunievics, 1996; Sykes, 1999; Toro-Alfonso, 1995; Xavier, 2000). Another example of discrimination is the enforcement of restrictive laws and policies which hinder their full enjoyment of rights and privileges, and limit their access to social services, marriage, parenting, and fair educational and employment opportunities, among other things (American Educational Gender Services, 2001; Harper & Schneider, 1999). In other words, their social vulnerability is directly related to their marginalization, prejudice, and lack of social and structural support.

In addition to these elements, the ignorance and *transphobia* that permeates society in general not only affect their quality of life but also influence how they are approached in prevention efforts. The scarcity of knowledge of this subject and the weak commitment to the transgender community both account for the lack of appropriate HIV/AIDS and other sexually transmitted disease preventive interventions among transgenders (Bockting, Robinson & Rosser, 1998).

Intervention efforts directed to the transgender community must be based on knowledge of the social and cultural factors that affect them. This is particularly relevant in Latino communities, where socialization depends on traditional cultural characteristics and values, which are promoted by social institutions' discourses.

Previous Studies with Transgenders in Puerto Rico

There have been few efforts directed to transgenders in the Puerto Rican context. The first one took place in 1995, when the Puerto Rico AIDS Foundation carried out an HIV prevention program with transgenders (Toro-Alfonso, 1995). Its main objective was to develop a description of the transgender population and identify risk factors for HIV infection. This effort included a gatekeeper from the transgender community. Participants were 19 MTF transgenders who reported all of the following: high levels of alcohol and other drug use, high levels of stress associated with sex work, discrimination, marginalization, and financial dependence on welfare.

Four years later, we (Rodríguez-Madera & Toro-Alfonso, 2000) developed a study to identify risk factors for HIV infection with a larger sample (50 MTF). The method implemented for this study and some of the results follow.

METHOD

For the purpose of this study we used a mixed method approach; specifically, a two-phase design which included a quantitative phase followed by a qualitative one (Tashakkoti & Teddle, 1998). For the first phase, we developed a quantitative questionnaire in order to obtain uniformity in specific information and to have an overview. For the qualitative phase, we used an interview guide to more deeply explore social discourses regarding gender construction.

Participants

Due to the sense of underground identities, it is hard to recruit willing participants from the transgender community. Therefore, we used a convenience sample. In exchange for a stipend, a gatekeeper (a MTF individual who has long been a leader and activist in the transgender community) agreed to help facilitate the recruitment process. After receiving training regarding the study's details, she informed participants about the nature of the research, what was expected of their participation, how to contact her or the principal investigator to obtain more information, and about participant financial incentive.

Description

A total of 50 MTF Puerto Rican transgenders participated in the study. Two of them participated in the interviews. Participants lived in the metropolitan area of San Juan. The average age was 27 years. The majority of them (74%) identified themselves as transsexuals, and 67% presented their gender identity openly (24 hours/7 days a week). None had undergone a sex change surgery, due to its cost and that being a "woman with penis" is his/her main attraction to "tricks."[1] This is important, considering that 74% worked in the sex industry.

Participants showed low levels of formal education: 35% did not finish high school and only 7% were able to go to college. They also informed a low income. Nearly half (41%) received less than 500 USD monthly. More than half (56%) showed high levels of alcohol and drug use.

Instruments

Quantitative Phase

We adapted an instrument developed by Corby & the State Office of AIDS (n.d.). The original version was in English and had been designed to be administered using a "face to face" format (Sykes, 1999). It included seven sections that asked about: (a) specific information regarding transgender population (Ex: sexual anatomy, gender identification), (b) socio-demographic data, (c) knowledge and attitude toward HIV, (d) sexual practices with main partners, (e) sexual practices with other partners, including amount and kind of partners, and (f) substance use.

Later, we developed a self-administered questionnaire in Spanish (Rodríguez-Madera & Toro-Alfonso, 1999). This version was submitted to an expert evaluation and followed by a pilot study. The final battery included a total of six questionnaires.

Qualitative Phase

We used the same *Socio-demographic Questionnaire* of the previous phase and developed a *Semi-structured Interview Guide*, which was evaluated by three experts who work in the area of gender and sexuality, with transgender populations, and are experienced in qualitative methodology.

Procedure and Analysis

We delivered the instruments, *Consent Information Form*, and the incentives (20 USD per participant) to the gatekeeper, who was in charge of the 50 participant recruitment. The administration of questionnaires spanned a three-month period. Once we had the instruments completed, we analyzed the data and generated frequencies and percentages using the Statistical Package for Social Science (SPSS) software.

After completing this process, we invited two participants for two-hour in-depth interviews, which were conducted the same week. We gave them a 50 USD incentive. Discourse analysis was made to the information gathered through interviews. For the purpose of this work, we focused our analysis on how gender discourses regarding the "feminine," specifically the ones related to aesthetic standards and sexual practices, can render MTF transgenders vulnerable to HIV infection.

RESULTS

Quantitative Phase

Most of the participants (92%) informed that they were born with a "masculine" sexual anatomy; the rest informed having an androgynous anatomy. Only 68% used the term "transgender" to describe themselves.

In terms of the HIV related information, 57% of the participants had knowledge of HIV modes of transmission but still engaged in high-risk sexual practices. They presented a low perception of risk for infection (59%). A total of 14% informed that they were HIV positive, 24% had never been tested for HIV, 62% of whom cited as their reason for not being tested that they felt sure of their seronegativity, and 18% have had another type of sexually transmitted disease (STD).

Almost half of the participants (45%) informed having made no behavioral change in order to protect themselves against HIV infection. Most of their unprotected sexual intercourse had been with primary partners, not with casual partners or "tricks." Figure 2 shows the amount of participants that had had sexual intercourse with primary partners, casual partners, and "tricks" during the last month; while Figure 3 presents the proportion of unprotected sex with these partners.

Many participants expressed being victims of all kinds of social barriers, such as prejudice and difficulties in accessing employment and social services, among others (Figure 4). Most felt that they had poor personal and institutional support networks. Specifically, 55% reported being victims of discrimination, 42% had difficulties obtaining government-based social services, and 60% showed an interest in gender counseling.

In terms of gender-related needs, we identified many instances in which these needs were imposed by social discourses regarding feminine gender roles, such as a woman's physical appearance. Participants' responses evidenced an aesthetic standard of the feminine, characterized by big breasts, wide hips, thinness, delicate facial features, and long hair, among others. Motivated by these social demands, 74% were using hormones from illegal markets, and 31% had undergone aesthetic surgeries in less expensive settings in South America. Most of them (89%) did not have medical follow up for hormone treatment or for surgeries.

Qualitative Phase

Sense of Being a Woman and Aesthetic Demands of Feminine Gender

Participants preferred to be identified as women rather than of transgendered people, and liked to be called by their "feminine" names. In fact, having a feminine name is apparently an important step in the process of gender construction. After the name, comes the body. That is why the body has to be congruent with gender identity (Gagné & Tewksbury, 1998), because it is through the body that people present themselves to others. But, even when body transformation can be a tortuous process, the sense of being a woman transcends corporeal issues (Quote 1):

> (1) I am a woman even if I have hair in my face . . . Even if I have a hairy body . . . Even if I have a penis. Even if I am sexually functional and I use my penis, I feel I am a woman.

This quote presents two important details regarding the "feminine." First, it is the assumption that feminine bodies are clean or hairless. This is a legacy of social discourses that establish rigid notions about how a woman's body should look. Second, it implies the "biological fact" that since women do not have a penis it is therefore not in their "sexual nature" to be sexually functional; meaning to penetrate their partner.

It is important to answer these questions. How are women's bodies? What is "natural" to women's bodies? What defines a "natural" woman's body? In patriarchal societies, and according to Derrida's conception of how opposites are defined in a binary system (Namaste,

FIGURE 2. Participants' Sexual Partners

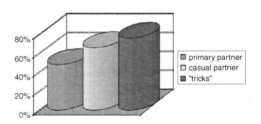

FIGURE 3. Unprotected Sex with Sexual Partners

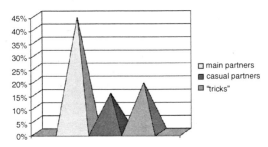

FIGURE 4. Social and Institutional Obstacles Identified by Participants

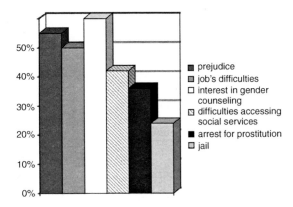

2000), a woman's body is the opposite of a man's. The answer to the above questions seems to be simply approached using sexual anatomy as the key factor. Thus, a woman's body is representative of motherhood and non-penetrative sexuality (Quote 2). This explains the emphasis on breasts and a vagina as the key elements of what it is to be a woman (Inciardi, Surrat, Telles, & Pok, 2001) (Quote 3).

> *(2) When I interact with my partner; a man, it provokes me . . . the desire of being a mother. Even if I know that I can not have children by myself, still this is the most important part for me [of being a woman].*

> *(3) In scientific terms, we categorize the thing in two ways: female because it has a vagina or male because it has a penis. In this sense, it [vagina] is the only thing that I do not have feminine. Because, I have breasts not because they make me feel more feminine, but because they help*

me to be accepted by the society. They help men to feel more comfortable for intimacy.

Interestingly, participants' discourses regarding the "feminine" evidenced another issue. They did place emphasis on breasts, but showed no interest in having a vagina. On the contrary, they cited the absence of a penis as "the characteristic" of the "feminine." This supports the assertion by some theorists that many MTF transgenders show repugnance for the vagina, and therefore find the sex change surgery unnecessary (Inciardi, Surrat, Telles, & Pok, 2001). This attitude may reflect a general devaluation of women, and specifically of the vagina as the symbol of women's biology, in this community. According to these authors, this issue suggests that MTF individuals tend to be socialized with the typical prejudice that men in patriarchal societies exhibit against women.

On the other hand, the "biological fact" that women do not have a penis seems to influence participants' perception of their own bodies. The negation of the penis are evident: "this part of me is like an arm, a leg . . . I have it, but I do not pay attention to it." This incongruence seems to be compensated by the overemphasis on the breasts, specifically because they symbolize womanhood and are a useful tool in catching a male's attention: "I move my breast when I want to get the attention of a man."

In many cases, the experience of being a MTF transgender requires an adjustment to gender binary demands. Thus, it turns into a fight to "pass" as a member of one gender or another without people noticing (Kammerer, Mason, Connors, & Durkee, 2001). The failure or success of "passing" not only depends on how a woman looks, but how women behave.

Women's Behavior: Social and Sexual Interaction

Other social discourses regarding the "feminine" that were present in participants' responses were related to the perpetuation of traditional gender roles, for example, the importance of motherhood, marriage, and specific characteristics socially attributed to women such as sensitivity, delicateness, emotional weakness, and passiveness, among others (Quote 4).

These characteristics are common, particularly within the context of patriarchal societies.

> *(4) To be a woman is being a sensitive person, spiritual and lovely. Even men can have some of these qualities, women have more.*

It seems that the social construction of the "feminine" has a strong impact not only on how participants perceive and construct their own bodies, but also on their sexual behavior. Traditionally, social discourses regarding feminine gender put women in a receptive role during sexual intercourse based on what is "natural" to their bodies. This assumption influences transgenders' sexual practices (Quote 5). It is clear that women's receptive sexual role not only tends to limit their sexual experiences, it also places women who want to transcend these notions in a questionable space. As we may see in the following comment, the possibility of a woman penetrating her sexual partner seems to be relegated to sex as an interchange of merchandise. Moreover, a receptive sexual role alludes to heterosexuality (Quote 6).

> *(5) I am always penetrated because I am a woman. There are people that make certain arrangements, but that is not my case. They do it for money. In the moment a man tries to approach me he knows what is going to happen in bed and he is not going to ask me something different because he knows that I am a woman!*

> *(6) I have sexual relationships from the perspective that I am a woman. I have breasts because it helps my partner to deal with my biological sex. Yes . . . The first thing that I show is a "tit." It is the hook. Sometimes they [partners] ask me: "Am I gay because I'm having sex with you?" And I ask: "Are you having sex with me because I have a penis or because I look like a woman? What did you see in me?" "You look like a woman." "Oh, so you can not say that you are gay because even if you are aware of my biological sex and enjoy that, you are with me because I look feminine. Because, if I had beard and look masculine . . . Will you do it? So, you are not gay."*

Having seen through this research that the tendency among the transgender community is to perpetuate traditional gender roles, the inevitable question is then, "What are the implications for MTF transgenders who construct a gender identity that places them in a vulnerable situation, particularly for HIV infection?" It seems a safe assumption that the sexual experience of an MTF who manifests this traditional, binary gender construction, regardless of his/her actual sexual anatomy, will be subject to the same vulnerability as that of a "biological woman." In other words, a MTF will most likely face the same difficulties that "biological" women face in practicing safer sex conducts. This explains the high HIV prevalence among MTF transgenders (Clements-Nolle, Marx, Guzman, & Katz, 2001; Sykes, 1999). Therefore, gender construction is an evident obstacle for HIV prevention.

DISCUSSION

The data gathered through this study evidences that the assumption by MTF transgenders of traditional female gender roles has to be considered as a factor that increases their vulnerability for HIV infection. Other important factors to consider include the daily experiences of prejudice, stigma, marginalization, lack of social support, and physical and emotional violence.

The difficulties women face in their negotiation for the practice of safer sex is based on the socially constructed inequalities of gender, not on their biology. One example of this is the fact that women tend not to protect themselves with their partners due to the way they construct and experience romantic love. This is one of the most serious difficulties in HIV prevention work (Ortiz-Torres, Serrano-García, & Torres-Burgos, 2000). Our findings support this notion. Participants in this study reported that they protect themselves more with "tricks" and casual partners than they do with their primary partner, as a result of their "feminine" gender socialization. Women often base their partnership on the values of truth, love, and trust. According to these values, many "biological women" adhere to the philosophy that if you trust your partner, you do not have to protect yourself. The same may be true for MTF transgenders.

In summary, the reproduction of social discourses regarding the "feminine" influences MTF transgenders' perception and construction of their bodies, their sexual behavior, and their interactions with other people. In addition, these social discourses lead them to ignore the existence of their penis because it breaks the female imaginary, which can negatively influence safer sex practices, specifically condom use. Having a penis may be considered a luxury in the sex industry because it is a turn on to "look like a chick with a dick," but we can not deny the sexual risks involved in "not paying attention to this part of the body."

Taking gender construction issues into consideration for HIV prevention is an important step in developing adequate strategies for the transgender population. We emphasize the importance of: (1) addressing gender construction in HIV preventative intervention, considering the way that feminine gender identity can present difficulties in the practice of safer sex, (2) approaching the issue based on the social discourses that prevail in specific socio-demographical contexts, and (3) developing exploratory studies with transgenders to obtain adequate information about their gender construction and including this subject in intervention goals.

In conclusion, we can not overlook important elements related to social vulnerability among transgenders such as lack of social and institutional support, among others. Furthermore, greater attention should be given to gender construction issues and their role in HIV prevention efforts designed for the MTF transgender community.

NOTE

1. Refers to clients in the sex industry.

REFERENCES

American Educational Gender Services. (2001). *Transgénero, ¿qué significa?* Access on August 20, 2001 at, *http://www.youthresource.com/espanol/librería/transgenero.htm.*

Bockting, W.O., & Kirk, S. (2001). Preface. In W. Bockting & S. Kirk (Eds.), *Transgender and HIV: Risks, prevention, and care* (pp. xix-xxiii). New York, NY: The Haworth Press, Inc.

Bockting, W., Rosser, B.R., & Scheltema, K. (1999). Transgender HIV prevention: Implementation and evaluation of a workshop. *Health Education Research: Theory and Practice, 14,* 177-183.

Bockting, W.O., Robinson, B.E., & Rosser, B.R. (1998). Transgender HIV prevention: A qualitative needs assessment. *AIDS Care, 10,* 505-26.

Butler, J. (1993). Bodies that matter. In J. Price & M. Shildrick (Eds.), *Feminist theory and the body* (pp. 235-45). New York, NY: Routledge.

Califia P. (1999). Love me gender. Access on July 12, 1999 at, *http://www.thebody.com/poz/features/10_99/html.*

Center for AIDS Prevention Studies. (2001). *What are the HIV prevention needs of male-to-female transgender persons (male-to-female)?* Access on September 9, 2001 at, *http://www.caps.ucsf.edu.maletofemale.html.*

Clements-Nolle, K., Marx, R., Guzman, R., & Katz, M. (2001). HIV prevalence, risk behaviors, health care use, and mental health status of transgender persons in San Francisco: Implications for public health intervention. *American Journal of Public Health, 91,* 915-21.

Collazo-Valentín, L.M. (1999). ¿Qué es la mujer? Revisión del signo mujer a través de las nociones sexo, género y rol. Unpublished Master Thesis, University of Puerto Rico. San Juan, PR.

Corby, N., & The State Office of AIDS. (n.d.). *Outreach Based HIV-Related Behavioral Surveillance.* Long Beach, CA: California State University.

Ettner, R. (1999). *Gender loving care.* New York, NY: W.W. Norton & Company.

Flecha, A. (2000). *Cuerpos en las fronteras: Violaciones feministas y visita a lo pornográfico.* Unpublished Master Thesis, University of Puerto Rico. San Juan, PR.

Gagné, P., & Tewksbury, R. (1998). Conformity pressures and gender resistance among transgendered individuals. *Social Problems, 45,* 80-101.

Harper, G., & Schneider, M. (1999). Giving lesbian, gay, bisexual, and transgendered people and communities a voice in community research action. *The Community Psychologist, 32,* 41-43.

Inciardi, J., Surrat, H., Telles, P., & Pok, B. (2001). Sex, drugs, and the culture of travestismo in Rio de Janeiro. In W. Bockting, & S. Kirk (Eds.), *Transgender and HIV: Risks, prevention, and care* (pp. 1-12). New York, NY.: The Haworth Press, Inc.

Kammerer, N., Mason, T., Connors, M., & Durkee, R. (2001). Transgender health and social service needs in the context of HIV risk. In *Transgender and HIV: Risks, prevention, and care* (pp. 39-57). New York, NY: The Haworth Press, Inc.

Lunievicz, J. (1996). Transgender positive. *Body positive, IX.* Access on August 20, 2001 at, *http://www.thebody.com/bp/nov96/transg/html.*

Nakano-Glenn, E. (1999). The social construction and institutionalization of gender and race: An integrative framework. In M. Marx Ferree, J. Lorber & B. Hess (Eds.), *Revisioning gender* (pp. 3-43). Thousand Oaks, CA: SAGE.

Namaste, V. (2000). *Invisible lives: The erasure of transsexuals and transgendered people*. Chicago, Ill: University Chicago Press.

Ortiz-Torres, B., Serrano-García, I., & Torres-Burgos, N. (2000). Subverting culture: Promoting HIV/AIDS prevention among Puerto Rican and Dominican women. *American Journal of Community Psychology, 28*, 859-82.

PASET. (2001). *HIV/AIDS Surveillance Report*. San Juan, PR: Department of Health.

Rodríguez-Madera, S., & Toro-Alfonso, J. (July, 2000). *The community we don't dare to mention: An exploratory study regarding social vulnerability, high risk sex conduct, and HIV/AIDS in Puerto Rico's transgender community*. Poster presented at XIII International AIDS Conference, Durban, South Africa.

Rodríguez-Madera, S., & Toro-Alfonso, J. (1999). *Social Vulnerability and High-risk Behavior for HIV Infection for Transgenders Questionnaire*. San Juan, PR: University Center for Psychological Research and Services, University of Puerto Rico.

Sykes, D.L. (1999). Transgendered people: An "invisible" population. *California HIV/AIDS Update, 12*, 82-5.

Tashakkori, A., & Teddlie, C. (1998). *Mixed methodology: Combining qualitative and quantitative approaches*. Thousand Oaks, CA: SAGE.

Toro-Alfonso, J. (1995). Trabajo en promoción de salud en una comunidad de trabajadores sexuales en San Juan (Puerto Rico) y la prevención del virus de immunodeficiencia adquirida (VIH/SIDA). *Avances en Psicología Clínica Latinoamericana, 13*, 55-70.

Vance, C. (1999). Anthropology rediscovers sexuality: A theoretical comment. In R. Parker & P. Aggleton (Eds.), *Culture, society and sexuality* (pp. 39-54). London, Eng.: UCL Press.

Varas Díaz, N. & Toro-Alfonso, J. (2001). A revision of HIV/AIDS public policy in Puerto Rico, Dominican Republic, Ecuador and Honduras: Tensions, limitations and achievements. *Interamerican Journal of Psychology, 35*, 113-132.

Wallach-Scott, J. (1999a). Gender as a useful category of historical analysis. In R. Parker & P. Aggleton (Eds.), *Culture, society and sexuality* (pp. 57-75). London, Eng.: UCL Press.

Xavier, J. (2000). *The Washington, DC transgender needs assessment survey*. Washington, DC: Gender Education and Advocacy.

Are Transgender Persons at Higher Risk for HIV Than Other Sexual Minorities? A Comparison of HIV Prevalence and Risks

Walter Bockting, PhD
Chiung-Yu Huang, PhD
Hua Ding, MPH
Beatrice "Bean" Robinson, PhD
B. R. Simon Rosser, PhD, MPH

SUMMARY. Recent studies have shown that transgender people are at high risk for HIV. Few studies, however, have directly compared the HIV risks and sexual health of transgender persons with that of other sexual minority populations. This study used baseline data of intervention studies targeting transgender persons, men who have sex with men, and women who have sex with women and men to compare their HIV risk behavior and sexual health. No significant differences were found between transgender persons and nontransgender men or women in consistent condom use or attitudes toward condom use. Transgender persons were less likely to have multiple partners and more likely to be monogamous than men who have sex with men; no differences were found between transgender persons and the women in this respect. When combining data on condom use, monogamy, and multiple partners, transgender persons did not differ from either nontransgender group in their overall risk for HIV. Transgender persons were less likely than the men or the women to have been tested for HIV. With regard to HIV prevalence, 17% of the men compared to only one transgender person and none of the women reported being HIV-positive. Transgender persons were also less likely than men who have sex with men to use drugs; no differences were found in the use of alcohol. However, with regard to mental health, transgender persons were more likely than the men to have experienced depression and more likely than men or women to have considered or attempted suicide. Finally, transgender persons reported the lowest levels of support from family and peers. Thus, in our sample, transgender persons appear to be at lower risk for HIV but at higher risk for mental health concerns than men who have sex with men. Remarkably few

Walter Bockting, PhD, and Beatrice "Bean" Robinson, PhD, are Associate Professors, and B. R. Simon Rosser, PhD, MPH, is Professor, all affiliated with the Program in Human Sexuality, Department of Family Medicine and Community Health, University of Minnesota Medical School. Chiung-Yu Huang, PhD, is Mathematical Statistician, Biostatistics Research Branch, National Institute of Allergy and Infectious Diseases, National Institutes of Health. Hua Ding, MPH, is Biostatistician, Department of Biostatistics, School of Medicine, Vanderbilt University.

Address correspondence to: Walter Bockting, PhD, Program in Human Sexuality, 1300 South Second Street, Suite 180, Minneapolis, MN 55454 USA (E-mail: bockt001@umn.edu).

The authors thank Anne Marie Weber-Main, PhD, for her critical review and editorial suggestions on earlier drafts of this manuscript.

This study was made possible through a grant from the Minnesota Department of Health, MDH/A23777.

[Haworth co-indexing entry note]: "Are Transgender Persons at Higher Risk for HIV Than Other Sexual Minorities? A Comparison of HIV Prevalence and Risks." Bockting, Walter et al. Co-published simultaneously in *International Journal of Transgenderism* (The Haworth Medical Press, an imprint of The Haworth Press, Inc.) Vol. 8, No. 2/3, 2005, pp. 123-131; and: *Transgender Health and HIV Prevention: Needs Assessment Studies from Transgender Communities Across the United States* (ed: Walter Bockting, and Eric Avery) The Haworth Medical Press, an imprint of The Haworth Press, Inc., 2005, pp. 123-131. Single or multiple copies of this article are available for a fee from The Haworth Document Delivery Service [1-800-HAWORTH, 9:00 a.m. - 5:00 p.m. (EST). E-mail address: docdelivery@haworthpress.com].

differences were found between transgender persons and women who have sex with women and men–a finding which might reflect the impact of social stigma on sexual health and have implications for the design of future HIV/STI prevention efforts. *[Article copies available for a fee from The Haworth Document Delivery Service: 1-800-HAWORTH. E-mail address: <docdelivery@haworthpress.com> Website: <http://www.HaworthPress.com> © 2005 by The Haworth Press, Inc. All rights reserved.]*

KEYWORDS. HIV risk, sexual health, transgender, MSM, bisexual women

INTRODUCTION

A steady increase has been observed in the number of research reports describing the HIV prevention and related health needs of the transgender population (Clements-Nolle et al., 2001; Kenagy, 2002; Nemoto et al., 2004). These studies indicate that, at least among certain subgroups, transgender people are at substantially high risk for HIV, with prevalence rates ranging from 19% to 35%. Some have argued that transgender persons might be at even greater risk of HIV infection and transmission than are men who have sex with men (Boles & Elifson, 1994; Nemoto et al., 1999; Xavier, 2005). The evidence for this, however, is not definitive. Most transgender needs assessments have relied on convenience samples, because it is difficult to obtain a representative sample of this hidden population. Thus, the reported risks might not be representative of the larger transgender population. Moreover, few studies have directly compared the risk behavior and sexual health of transgender persons to that of other sexual minority populations recruited in similar ways from similar environments.

To our knowledge, only two studies have directly compared the HIV prevention and health needs of transgender persons with those of other at risk populations. Nemoto and colleagues (1999) interviewed three groups: male-to-female transgenders (n = 25), homosexual and bisexual men (n = 122), and heterosexual women (n = 26). Transgender persons reported the greatest number of sexual partners. Transgender persons and heterosexual women were more likely to inject drugs than were the men, and less likely to be tested for HIV. No group differences were found in attitudes toward condom use. The HIV seroprevalence rate was high across all three groups (41-60% of those tested), though this might be explained, at least in part, by the fact that participants were recruited from AIDS service organizations in a high prevalence area (San Francisco).

In research with nonclinical samples, Mathy (2001) compared the relationship status and mental health of 73 transgender persons to that of several different samples of nontransgender women and men, either homo- or heterosexual. For the majority of measures, transgender persons were most similar to lesbian women and different from all other groups. Nearly identical proportions of transgender persons and lesbian women were either married or in a faithfully committed relationship, whereas homosexual men were significantly less likely than transgender persons and lesbian women to be married or in a committed relationship. Transgender persons were more likely to take medications for a psychiatric condition and more likely to have a problem with alcohol than were nontransgender men and heterosexual women, but no differences were found between transgender persons and lesbian women in these respects. For the latter two groups, the author attributed their higher likelihood of mental health and substance abuse problems to their experiencing the double stigma of gender (transgender or woman) and sexual orientation (lesbian, gay, or bisexual, since most transgender persons did not identify as heterosexual).

In Mathy's (2001) study, not all transgender persons were recruited in the same manner as the comparison groups. Also, in both previous studies (Nemoto et al., 1999; Mathy, 2001), the sample size of transgender persons was small, limiting the interpretation and generalizability of findings. At the University of Minnesota Program in Human Sexuality, we had a unique opportunity to conduct larger group comparisons among different sexual minority groups. Since 1997, we have been conducting and evaluating a sexual health approach to HIV prevention that targets transgender persons, men who have sex with men, and women who have sex with women and men (Bockting et al., 2005; Robinson et al., 2002; Rosser et al., 2002). Although the specific content of the intervention differs for each target population, each version of the intervention shares a similar conceptual underpinning and format. In addition, participants across the three comparison groups are recruited with similar methods from the same area of Minnesota, a low HIV prevalence state (Centers for Disease Control and Prevention, 2003). This article reports our comparison of the HIV prevalence, HIV risk behaviors, and sexual health of these three sexual minority groups (total sample N = 809). Data were acquired from a questionnaire completed by participants just prior to participating in a sexual health seminar. On the basis of the research reviewed above, along with our clinical experience with members of the three target populations, we expected transgender persons to report the highest levels of HIV prevalence and risk behavior, followed by men who have sex with men, and women who have sex with women and men. In addition, we expected transgender persons to be the least likely to have ever had an HIV test, to have the highest levels of depression, suicidal ideation, and substance abuse, to have the least positive attitudes toward condom use (due to genital dysphoria), and to report the lowest levels of family and peer support.

METHODS

Participants

Participants were persons aged 18 years and older recruited between 1997 and 2002 from across Minnesota to participate in a two-day sexual health seminar. Although the content of the seminar differed by target population, participants across the three comparison groups were recruited from the same GLBT (gay, lesbian, bisexual, and transgender) community in the same geographic area and by similar methods–brochures, community newspaper advertisements, postings on the Internet, environmental outreach, and health providers. Because seminars were offered more than once to each

target population, anyone who had previously attended a seminar in the last two years was excluded from data analysis. This resulted in a total of 809 participants for this analysis: 207 transgender (TG) persons (77% male-to-female, 23% female-to-male), 480 men who have sex with men (MSM), and 122 women who have sex with women and men (WSWM). We chose to regard transgender persons as a single group rather than distinguish between male-to-females and female-to-males, because both transcend gender and face associated social challenges, and because previous research with a sample drawn from the same study population revealed few significant differences in HIV risks and sexual health between male-to-females and female-to-males (Bockting et al., 2005). Table 1 presents the demographic characteristics of the three groups.

Instruments

Participants completed a paper-and-pencil questionnaire immediately prior to participating in the seminar. The questionnaire assessed demographics (age, education, income, ethnicity, religion), sexual identity, HIV risk behavior (four components), and the following sexual health variables: physical and mental health, alcohol and drug use, attitudes toward condom use, and social (peer and family) support.

Four components of HIV risk behaviors (Table 2) were assessed (Hines et al., 1998):

1. *Condom use* was measured with five items that asked participants if and how often they used condoms during anal or vaginal intercourse with their primary or other partner(s) during the last three months (Rosser et al., 2002). Responses were dichotomized to represent inconsistent condom use (condom not used every time) versus consistent condom use (condom used every time). Participants who reported no anal or vaginal intercourse during the last three months were excluded.

2. *Number of sexual partners* was assessed with three items asking participants how many sexual partners they had and if they had anal or vaginal intercourse with their primary and/or other partners in the

last three months (Rosser et al., 2002). Responses were dichotomized into one sexual partner and multiple (more than one) partners. Participants who reported no anal or vaginal intercourse in the last three months were excluded.

3. *Relationship monogamy* was assessed using the sexual partner items and two additional items that asked participants if they were in a primary sexual relationship and whether or not this relationship was open or closed (Rosser et al., 2002). Responses were dichotomized into monogamous (one partner and relationship closed) and non-monogamous (one partner and relationship open or multiple partners). Participants who reported no anal or vaginal intercourse during the last three months were excluded.

4. *Overall level of sexual risk* was assessed by combining consistent condom use and monogamy. Responses were dichotomi-

zed into low risk (monogamy and consistent condom use, monogamy and inconsistent condom use, non-monogamy and consistent condom use, or no anal or vaginal intercourse in the last three months) and high risk (non-monogamy and inconsistent condom use).

Each of the sexual health variables in Table 3 was assessed with a single item. Participants were asked if they ever had an HIV test and if they had been diagnosed with HIV or AIDS. Depression was assessed by the question: "*In the past year* have you had *two consecutive weeks or more* during which you felt sad, blue, or depressed; or when you lost interest or pleasure in things that you usually cared about or enjoyed?" In addition, participants were asked if they had considered or attempted suicide in the last three years.

Consuming five or more alcoholic drinks in one sitting in the last two weeks was used as an

TABLE 1. Demographics of study sample ($N = 809$) by sexual minority group.

Variable	Transgender persons ($N = 207$)	Men who have sex with men ($N = 480$)	Women who have sex with women and men ($N = 122$)	p[3]
	Mean *(SD)*			
Age (years)	40.8 (11.4)	37.5 (10.1)	33.1 (10.4)	< .0001
	n (%)			
Education				< .001
High school	31 (16%)	34 (8%)	4 (3%)	
Some college, vocational school	83 (42%)	149 (34%)	32 (26%)	
College graduate, graduate/ professional school	86 (43%)	358 (59%)	85 (70%)	
Income[1]				< .001
Below poverty level	43 (22%)	64 (14%)	8 (7%)	
Above poverty level	149 (78%)	396 (86%)	108 (93%)	
Ethnicity				< .001
White	182 (92%)	352 (74%)	98 (82%)	
Of color	16 (8%)	121 (26%)	22 (18%)	
Religion				< .001
Catholic	14 (7%)	88 (19%)	8 (7%)	
Protestant	76 (40%)	209 (46%)	35 (30%)	
Atheist	35 (18%)	61 (13%)	8 (15%)	
Other	66 (35%)	101 (22%)	57 (48%)	
Relationship status[2]				< .0001
Primary partner	87 (48%)	138 (32%)	58 (78%)	
No primary partner	93 (52%)	299 (68%)	16 (32%)	

[1]Income level was assessed by a single item. Participants were classified as impoverished or not on the basis of U.S. Department of Health and Human Services 2002 poverty guidelines (U.S. DHHS, 2002).
[2]Participants who indicated being unsure whether or not they were in a primary relationship were coded as missing.
[3]Differences between groups were tested using ANOVA and Chi-square for independent samples.

TABLE 2. Comparison of HIV risk behaviors (past three months) in three sexual minority groups: transgender persons (TG), men who have sex with men (MSM), and women who have sex with women and men (WSWM). Sample *N* = 809.

Variable	n (%)			P-Value[1]	Odds Ratio (95% CI)		
	TG	MSM	WSWM		TG vs. MSM	TG vs. WSWM	MSM vs. WSWM
Inconsistent condom use	62 (63%)	179 (54%)	45 (68%)	n.s.			
Multiple partners	34 (34%)	209 (63%)	28 (42%)	< .0001	.33 (.20-.53)	n.s.	2.3 (1.3-4.0)
Nonmonogamy	60 (68%)	249 (80%)	43 (72%)	< .05	.47 (.27-.82)	n.s.	n.s.
Overall high risk	38 (20%)	132 (29%)	28 (24%)	n.s.			

[1]After controlling for Age and Education using logistic regression

TABLE 3. Comparison of sexual health variables in three sexual minority groups: transgender persons (TG), men who have sex with men (MSM), and women who have sex with women and men (WSWM). Sample *N* = 809.

Variable	n (%)			P-Value	Odds Ratio (95% CI)		
	TG	MSM	WSWM		TG vs. MSM	TG vs. WSWM	MSM vs. WSWM
HIV test ever	118 (60%)	408 (86%)	85 (70%)	< .0001	.25 (.16-.37)	.6 (.35-.99)	2.4 (1.5-3.9)
Depression	104 (52%)	182 (38%)	46 (40%)	< .05	1.6 (1.1-2.3)	n.s.	n.s.
Suicide[1]	95 (47%)	146 (31%)	38 (32%)	< .01	1.9 (1.3-2.7)	1.9 (1.2-3.2)	n.s.
Alcohol abuse	45 (20%)	142 (30%)	19 (16%)	< .01	n.s.	n.s.	2.4 (1.4-4.0)
Marijuana use	32 (16%)	125 (26%)	29 (24%)	= .01	.51 (.32-.80)	n.s.	n.s.
Other drug use	7 (3%)	45 (9%)	2 (2%)	= .001	.31 (.13-.75)	n.s.	7.8 (1.8-33.0)
Sexual problem due to substance use	22 (12%)	120 (25%)	18 (16%)	< .01	.33 (.20-.56)	n.s.	n.s.
	Mean (SD)				Mean Difference[5] (95% CI)		
Attitudes toward condom use[2]	3.6 (.78)	3.7 (.70)	3.8 (.63)	n.s.			
Peer contact[3]	2.0 (1.18)	3.0 (1.12)	2.1 (1.08)	< .0001	1.1 (.7-1.2)	n.s.	1.1 (.7-1.2)
Family support[4]	2.6 (1.53)	3.1 (1.38)	4.1 (1.83)	< .001	.5 (.2-.9)	1.4 (.9-1.9)	.9 (.4-1.3)

[1]Considered or attempted suicide in the last 3 years.
[2]Assessed on a 5-point Likert scale where 1 = strongly disagree and 5 = strongly agree. Higher scores indicate more positive attitudes.
[3]Assessed on a 5-point Likert scale where 1 = no social time spent with peers and 5 = all of social time spent with peers
[4]Assessed on a 5-point Likert scale where 1 = not at all supportive and 5 = very much supportive
[5]Mean difference after controlling for age and education. Only significant differences are reported based on p-values adjusted using Tukey's method.

indicator of alcohol abuse. The number of times marijuana or other drugs (e.g., cocaine, heroin, amphetamines, barbiturates) were used in the last three months was dichotomized into "any use" or "no use" of these substances. In addition, participants were asked if they had a sexual functioning problem caused by drinking or taking drugs.

Attitudes toward condom use were measured using a five-item scale adapted from Ross (1988). Each item was scored on a five-point Likert scale ranging from 1 = strongly disagree to 5 = strongly agree. Examples include "Condoms are good protection against STDs" and "I have a responsibility to use condoms during intercourse." Mean scores were calculated by converting negative items and by dividing the total scale score by the number of items completed. Thus, a higher mean score reflects a more positive attitude. Only scores from participants who completed all five attitude items were included in the analysis.

Contact with peers in one's sexual minority group (TG, MSM, or WSWM) was assessed by a single item asking participants to rate, on a five-point Likert scale, the portion of their social time spent with peers (1 = none, 5 = all the time). Family support was also assessed using a five-point Likert scale. Participants rated how supportive they felt their family members (parents and/or siblings) were regarding their sexual identity (1 = not at all supportive, 5 = very much supportive), with an option of "not applicable" for those who had not disclosed their identity to family members.

Procedure

Upon arrival at the seminar site (at community-based organizations, health clubs, or clinics already frequented by the target populations), participants gave informed consent to take part in an evaluation study of the intervention and completed a paper-and-pencil questionnaire prior to the start of the seminar. Each participant received a unique identifier (a code number) to protect confidentiality. This questionnaire took 20-30 minutes to complete. Participants also completed a post and 3-month follow-up questionnaire, but only data from the pre-seminar questionnaires were used in the analyses for this report. Two of the groups–transgender persons, and women who have sex with women and men–were offered no compensation due to a lack of funds; men who have sex with men received $20 upon completion of the post-test following the intervention.

Analysis

Statistical analyses were performed using SAS version 8.0 (SAS Institute, Inc., Gary, NC). We compared the distribution of age, education, income, ethnicity, and religion in the three sexual minority groups using ANOVA and Chi-square for independent samples (Table 1). The three groups differed significantly on each of these demographic variables. We chose to control for age and education in the subsequent analyses, because we expected age and education (and not ethnicity or religion) to differentially affect the three groups on the dependent variables of interest. We chose not to control for income because of its association

with age and education, and because the definition and measurement of income was less comparable across groups. Regression analyses were performed using SAS GLM procedure for continuous response variables and SAS LOGISTIC procedure for dichotomous response variables. In each regression model, we used age, education, and two dummy variables for the gender groups as covariates. Finally, we computed odds ratios (with 95% confidence intervals) for pair-wise gender group comparisons in dichotomous response variables and mean differences (with 95% confidence intervals) for continuous response variables. Significance level was set at .05.

RESULTS

Table 1 compares the demographics of the three sexual minority groups. Transgender persons reported the lowest levels of education and income; 22% of transgender participants had an income below the poverty level. About half of transgender participants reported having a primary sexual partner, compared to about one-third of men who have sex with men and 78% of the women who have sex with women and men.

Tables 2 and 3 compare the HIV risk behaviors and other sexual health variables, respectively, of the three sexual minority groups. After controlling for group differences in age and education, no significant differences were found between transgender persons and nontransgender men or women in consistent condom use (Table 2) or attitudes toward condom use (Table 3). As indicated by the data in Table 2, transgender persons were 3.1 times less likely than MSM to have multiple partners (95% CI = 1.9-5.0) and 2.1 times more likely than the men to be monogamous (95% CI = 1.2-3.7). No significant differences in these HIV risk behaviors were found between transgender persons and women who have sex with women and men. When combining data on condom use, monogamy, and multiple partners, transgender persons did not differ from nontransgender men or women in their overall risk for HIV.

As indicated by the data in Table 3, transgender persons were 4.1 (95% CI = 2.7-6.1) times less likely than MSM and 1.8 (95% CI =

1.01-3.0) times less likely than WSWM to have been tested for HIV; 17% of the MSM in our sample reported being HIV-positive, compared to only one transgender person and none of the WSWM. In terms of substance use, transgender persons were 2.0 (95% CI = 1.3-3.1) times less likely to smoke marijuana and 3.2 (95% CI = 1.3-7.7) times less likely to use other drugs than the men; transgender persons did not differ from men and women in the use of alcohol. Transgender persons were 3.0 (95% CI = 1.8-5.1) times less likely than the men to report a sexual functioning problem caused by alcohol or drugs.

In terms of mental health, transgender persons were 1.6 (95% CI = 1.1-2.3) times more likely than the men to have experienced depression and 1.9 (95% CI = 1.3-2.7) times more likely than either the men or women to have considered or attempted suicide. Transgender persons reported less contact with their peers than did the men (p < .0001) and less support from family than did either the men (p = .0001) or the women (p < .0001) in our sample.

DISCUSSION

This study compared the HIV prevalence and risks of transgender persons, men who have sex with men, and women who have sex with women and men in order to explore gender-based differences between these three sexual minority populations. Such differences will have implications for targeting HIV prevention efforts to specific subgroups of the gay, lesbian, bisexual, and transgender community. On the basis of previous research (Mathy, 2001; Nemoto et al., 1999), we expected transgender persons to report the highest levels of HIV prevalence and risk behavior, followed by the nontransgender men and the bisexually-active women. Our results, however, show a somewhat different picture.

First, our findings suggest that the high HIV prevalence found among certain subgroups of the transgender population (19% to 35%, e.g., Nemoto et al., 2004) may not be generalizable to the entire, or even the majority of this population. Among our participants–all of whom were recruited for intervention studies in a low-prevalence, primarily Caucasian state–only one of 207 transgender persons reported being

HIV-positive. (Of course, more of them could be HIV-positive but not know it, due to not having been tested for HIV [Clements-Nolle et al., 2001]). The higher HIV prevalence and risks found in other studies could be affected by risk cofactors such as low socioeconomic status and sex work, exacerbated by the double stigma associated with transgender and ethnic minority status (Bockting et al., 1998). The process by which transgender identity intersects with these structural risk factors deserves further study.

Second, we found no differences between the three sexual minority groups in attitudes toward condoms and our measure of *overall* HIV risk. This suggests that, when the context of unprotected sex is taken into account (e.g., inconsistent condom use within a monogamous relationship is low risk), the HIV risk of transgender persons is comparable to that of other sexual minority populations requiring targeted prevention.

Third, when we examined the various components of HIV risk behavior, transgender persons were actually *less* likely to report multiple partners and nonmonogamy than were MSM, though no difference was found between transgender persons (77% of whom were male-to-female) and WSWM. These findings are consistent with studies among gay, lesbian, bisexual, and transgender youth showing that males are more likely than females to have multiple partners and are less likely than females to be in a monogamous relationship (Lindley et al., 2003; Newman et al., 2000; Rotheram et al., 1999). Our results for these two measures support the hypotheses that (1) mechanisms of HIV risk differ by gender, and (2) transgender persons and nontransgender women who practice serial monogamy might be at risk primarily through the risk behavior of their male partners (Bockting et al., 2004; Newman et al., 2000). Therefore, interventions should empower transgender and nontransgender women to negotiate safer sex with their male partners. Moreover, HIV prevention efforts targeting men who have sex with women (heterosexually-identified or not) are urgently needed, including interventions that confront infidelity, homophobia, and compulsive sexual behavior (Bockting et al., 2004).

Our research with these populations included an assessment of other components of sexual health, specifically, drug use, alcohol abuse, mental health, and family/peer support–all potential cofactors of HIV risk. Drug use (not including marijuana) among the sample was low (2-9%), but most prevalent among MSM. This is in contrast to Nemoto's (1999) findings that transgender persons were twice as likely (28%) as MSM (13%) to have engaged in injection drug use. This discrepancy is likely due to the bias associated with convenience sampling. An interesting finding from our study is that some participants reported sexual functioning problems due to substance use. Sexual functioning problems have been associated with unsafe sex among African American women (Robinson et al., in press). Future research should explore how substance use impacts sexual functioning, and in turn, whether sexual functioning problems (such as erectile dysfunction) contribute to inconsistent condom use.

With regard to mental health, transgender persons were *more* likely to report depression than MSM and *more* likely to report suicidal ideation and attempts than the nontransgender men or women. Previous research has found high rates of depression and suicidal ideation or attempts among the transgender population (e.g., Clements-Nolle, 2001; Kenagy, 2005; Kenagy & Bostwick, 2005). Our results are also consistent with Mathy's (2001) findings and interpretation that transgender persons and lesbian women may have greater mental health problems than MSM as a result of experiencing the double stigma of gender and sexual orientation. The role of stigma in the mental health and HIV risk of transgender as well as other sexual minorities deserves further study (see also Meyer, 2003).

Transgender persons reported the lowest levels of family support of all three groups. WSWM reported higher levels of family support than MSM, which suggests that male homosexuality is more stigmatized than female homosexuality. However, MSM reported more peer support than the two other groups. Peer support may serve as a buffer to a lack of family acceptance (Frable et al., 1997), a buffer that our findings suggest is less available to transgender persons. Hence, transgender persons appear to be the most socially isolated of these three sex-

ual minority groups. Research has begun to establish a relationship between support of transgender identity by family and friends and mental health (Nuttbrock et al., 2002). The development of peer support for transgender persons, as well as bisexual women, could be an important asset in promoting their resilience and sexual health.

Our results should be interpreted cautiously in light of study limitations. Although recruitment was similar across the three sexual minority groups, we still relied on convenience samples. Therefore, the extent to which our findings are generalizable beyond the seminar participants is unclear. Also, we did not distinguish between male-to-female and female-to-male transgender persons. Although we controlled for differences in age and education, some of the observed differences could be due to the ethnic or religious differences between the three groups. Nevertheless, because all participants were recruited from the same community with very similar strategies and for the same purpose, we believe that the observed differences between the three groups are, at least in part, due to differences in their sexual identity. Another strength of our descriptive study is its use of comparison groups, allowing us to present the data gathered from transgender participants in the perspective of a known high risk group (men who have sex with men) and a group of bisexually-active women that, like transgender persons, lack a cohesive community where they can find consistent peer support.

In conclusion, the gay, lesbian, bisexual, and transgender community is diverse, and important differences exist in HIV risk factors and cofactors and corresponding prevention needs. Our findings indicate that men who have sex with men are the most likely to practice non-monogamy and have multiple sexual partners, whereas no differences were found in these risk factors between transgender persons and women who have sex with women and men. Of the three groups, transgender persons are the most likely to be depressed and at risk for suicide, and have the lowest level of social support. Future research should identify the social, psychological, and biological factors that account for these differences, and increase our understanding of how gender and sexual minority status affect sexual health.

REFERENCES

Bockting, W., Miner M., and Rosser, S. (2004). Male partners of transgender persons and HIV/STI risk: Findings from an Internet study of Latino men who have sex with men. Manuscript submitted for publication.

Bockting, W.O., Robinson, B.E., Forberg, J., and Scheltema, K. (2005). Evaluation of a sexual health approach to reducing HIV/STD risk in the transgender community. *AIDS Care, 17*(3), 289-303.

Bockting, W.O., Rosser, B.R.S., and Robinson, B.E. (1998). Transgender HIV prevention: A qualitative needs assessment. *AIDS Care, 10*(4), 505-526.

Boles, J., & Elifson, K.W. (1994). The social organization of transvestite prostitution and AIDS. *Social Science and Medicine, 39*(1), 85-93.

Centers for Disease Control and Prevention (2003). *HIV/ AIDS surveillance report, 15.* Atlanta, Georgia: US Department of Health and Human Services, Centers for Disease Control and Prevention. [Available at www.cdc.gov/hiv/stats/hasrlink.htm].

Clements-Nolle, K., Marx, R., Guzman, R., and Katz, M. (2001). HIV prevalence, risk behaviors, health care use, and mental health status of transgender persons: Implications for public health intervention. *American Journal of Public Health, 91*(6), 915-921.

Frable, D.E.S., Wortman, C., and Joseph, J. (1997). Predicting self esteem, well-being, and distress in a cohort of gay men: The importance of cultural stigma, personal visibility, community networks, and positive identity. *Journal of Personality, 65,* 599-624.

Hines, A.M., Snowden, L.R., and Graves, K.L. (1998). Acculturation, alcohol consumption and AIDS-related risky sexual behavior among African American women. *Women & Health, 27*(3), 17-35.

Kenagy, G.P. (2002). HIV among transgendered people. *AIDS Care, 14*(1), 127-134.

Kenagy, G.P. (2005). The health and social service needs of transgender people in Philadelphia. *International Journal of Transgenderism 8*(2/3), 49-56.

Kenagy, G.P. and Bostwick, W.B. (2005). Health and social service needs of transgender people in Chicago. *International Journal of Transgenderism 8*(2/3), 57-66.

Lindley, L.L., Nicholson, T.J., Kerby, M.B., and Lu, N. (2003). HIV/STI associated risk behaviors among self-identified lesbian, gay, bisexual, and transgender college students in the United States. *AIDS Education and Prevention, 15*(5), 413-429.

Mathy, R.M. (2001). A nonclinical comparison of transgender identity and sexual orientation: A framework for multicultural competence. *Journal of Psychology and Human Sexuality, 13*(1), 31-54.

Meyer, I.H. (2003). Prejudice, social stress, and mental health in lesbian, gay, and bisexual populations: Conceptual issues and research evidence. *Psychological Bulletin, 129*(5), 674-697.

Nemoto, T., Luke, D., Mamo, L., Ching, A., and Patria, J. (1999). HIV risk behaviours among male-to-female transgenders in comparison with homosexual and bisexual males and heterosexual females. *AIDS Care, 11*(3), 297-312.

Nemoto, T., Operario, D., Keatley, J., Han, L., and Soma, T. (2004). HIV risk behaviors among male-to-female transgender persons of color in San Francisco. *American Journal of Public Health, 94*(7), 1193-1199.

Newman, P.A. and Zimmerman, M.A. (2000). Gender differences in HIV-related sexual risk behavior among urban African American youth: A multivariate approach. *AIDS Education and Prevention, 12*(4), 308-325.

Nuttbrock, L., Rosenblum, A., and Blumenstein, R. (2002). Transgender identity affirmation and mental health. *International Journal of Transgenderism, 6*(4). [Available at www.symposion.com/ijt].

Robinson, B.E., Bockting, W.O., Rosser, B.R.S., Miner, M., and Coleman, E. (2002). The Sexual Health Model: Application of a sexological approach to HIV prevention. *Health Education Research; Theory and Practice, 17*(1), 43-57.

Robinson, B.E., Scheltema, K., and Cherry, T. (in press). Risky sexual behavior in low-income African American women: The impact of sexuality and acculturation. *Journal of Sex Research.*

Ross, M.W. (1988). Attitudes toward condoms as AIDS prophylaxis in homosexual men: Dimensions and measurement. *Psychology and Health, 2,* 291-299.

Rosser, B.R.S., Bockting, W.O., Rugg, D.L., Robinson, B.E., Ross, M.W., Bauer, G.R., and Coleman, E. (2002). A randomized controlled intervention trial of a sexual health approach to long-term HIV risk reduction for men who have sex with men: Effects of the intervention on unsafe sexual behavior. *AIDS Education and Prevention, 14,* Supplement A, 59-71.

Rotheram-Borus, M.J., Marelich, W.D., and Srinivasan, S. (1999). HIV risk among homosexual, bisexual, and heterosexual male and female youths. *Archives of Sexual Behavior, 28*(2), 159-177.

U.S. Department of Health and Human Services, Office of the Assistant Secretary for Planning and Evaluation (2002). *The 2002 HHS poverty guidelines.* [Available online at www.aspe.hhs.gov/poverty/02poverty.htm].

Xavier, J.M., Bobbin, M., Singer, B., and Budd, E. (2005). A needs assessment of transgendered people of color living in Washington, DC. *International Journal of Transgenderism, 8*(2/3), 31-47.

Index

Internet, 84
ISU. *See* Injection silicone use (ISU)

Jackson, M., xi-xiii,1
Jenkins, A., xiii,1
JSI Research & Training Institute, Inc., 65,76

Kammerer, N., 115
Keatley, J., 5
Kenagy, G.P., 2,49,57

Landers, S., 75
Lawrence, S., 75
Lombardi, E.L., 7
Lurie, S., 2,93

Male sexual partners, role in HIV infection among
    MtF transgender persons, 21-30. *See also*
    Male-to-female (MtF) transgender persons,
    HIV infection among, male sexual partners in
Male-to-female (MtF), defined, 95
Male-to-female (MtF) transgender persons, 6
    of color in San Francisco, health and social services
        for, 5-19. *See also* Transgender persons, of
        color in San Francisco, MtF, health and
        social services for
    HIV/AIDS prevention in, 113-122. *See also* HIV/
        AIDS prevention, in MtF transgender persons
        in Houston, Texas
    HIV infection among, 72-73
        introduction to, 68
        sex, drugs, violence, and HIV status among,
            67-74
            study of
                alcohol and drug use, 70,71t
                characteristics in, 69,69t
                data analysis in, 69
                discussion of, 72-73
                field notes in, 69,69t,71-72,71t
                methods in, 68-69
                partner violence in, 72
                procedure in, 68-69
                results of, 69-72,69t-71t
                sample in, 68,69,69t
                sexual behavior in, 70-71,71t
                STDs with HIV infection, 69-70,70t
                suicidal ideation in, 72
                survey instrument in, 68
    local responses to public health needs of, 6-7
Male-to-female (MtF) transgendered persons
    HIV infection among, male sexual partners and,
        21-30
        introduction to, 22-23
        study of

analysis of, 24,25
discussion of, 28-29
focus groups in, 24
instruments in, 23-25
limitations of, 28
methods in, 23-25,23t
participants in, 23,23t,24-25
procedure of, 24,25
results of, 25-28,25t-27t
male sexual partners of, interviews with, 23-24,23t
Mason, T., 115
Massachusetts Department of Public Health (MDPH),
    76
Mathy, R.M., 124
McCurdy, S., 67
MDPH. *See* Massachusetts Department of Public
    Health (MDPH)
Medicaid, 65
"Medical Care of Transgendered Patients," 109
Mental health issues, of transgender persons in Boston,
    82-83
Michael Callen–Audre Lorde Community Health
    Center, 109
MtF. *See* Male-to-female (MtF)

National Coalition of Anti-Violence Programs
    (NCAVP), 34
National Health Interview Survey, 59
National HIV/AIDS Clinician Consultation Center,
    108
National Institutes of Health, 108
National Resource Center, of AIDS Education and
    Training Center, 108
NCAVP. *See* National Coalition of Anti-Violence
    Programs (NCAVP)
Needle use, among transgender persons in Chicago, 62
Needs assessment
    in Boston, for access to health care for transgender
        persons in, 75-91
    of transgender persons
        in Boston, for access to health care. *See also*
            Transgender persons, health care for, access
            to, needs assessment in Boston study of
        of color in Washington, D.C., 31-47. *See also*
            Transgender persons, of color in Washington,
            D.C., needs assessment of
Nemoto, T., 1,5,124,130

Operario, D., 5

Packer, T., 21
Padgett, P., 67
Partner violence, among MtF transgender persons in
    Houston, Texas, 72

BOOK ORDER FORM!

Order a copy of this book with this form or online at:
http://www.haworthpress.com/store/product.asp?sku=5670

Transgender Health and HIV Prevention
Needs Assessment Studies
from Transgender Communities Across the United States

___ in softbound at $34.95 ISBN-13: 978-0-7890-3015-3 / ISBN-10: 0-7890-3015-2.

COST OF BOOKS _____

POSTAGE & HANDLING _____
US: $4.00 for first book & $1.50
for each additional book
Outside US: $5.00 for first book
& $2.00 for each additional book.

SUBTOTAL _____

In Canada: add 7% GST. _____

STATE TAX _____
CA, IL, IN, MN, NJ, NY, OH, PA & SD residents
please add appropriate local sales tax.

FINAL TOTAL _____
If paying in Canadian funds, convert
using the current exchange rate,
UNESCO coupons welcome.

☐ BILL ME LATER:
Bill-me option is good on US/Canada/
Mexico orders only; not good to jobbers,
wholesalers, or subscription agencies.

☐ Signature _____

☐ Payment Enclosed: $ _____

☐ PLEASE CHARGE TO MY CREDIT CARD:
☐ Visa ☐ MasterCard ☐ AmEx ☐ Discover
☐ Diner's Club ☐ Eurocard ☐ JCB

Account # _____

Exp Date _____

Signature _____
(Prices in US dollars and subject to change without notice.)

PLEASE PRINT ALL INFORMATION OR ATTACH YOUR BUSINESS CARD

Name

Address

City   State/Province   Zip/Postal Code

Country

Tel   Fax

E-Mail

May we use your e-mail address for confirmations and other types of information? ☐ Yes ☐ No We appreciate receiving
your e-mail address. Haworth would like to e-mail special discount offers to you, as a preferred customer.
We will never share, rent, or exchange your e-mail address. We regard such actions as an invasion of your privacy.

Order from your **local bookstore** or directly from
The Haworth Press, Inc. 10 Alice Street, Binghamton, New York 13904-1580 • USA
Call our toll-free number (1-800-429-6784) / Outside US/Canada: (607) 722-5857
Fax: 1-800-895-0582 / Outside US/Canada: (607) 771-0012
E-mail your order to us: orders@haworthpress.com

For orders outside US and Canada, you may wish to order through your local
sales representative, distributor, or bookseller.
For information, see http://haworthpress.com/distributors

(Discounts are available for individual orders in US and Canada only, not booksellers/distributors.)
Please photocopy this form for your personal use.
www.HaworthPress.com

The Haworth Press Inc.

BOF05